Tears of Gethsemane

A Pastor's Journey through Leukemia

Sandra & Preston,

Your journey has been long and God's comfort amazing. May this book bring strength and courage for the rest of your journey.

Phil 4:12-13

Earl

Earl J. Spivey Jr.

ISBN 978-1-64569-727-5 (paperback)
ISBN 978-1-0980-0886-4 (hardcover)
ISBN 978-1-64569-728-2 (digital)

Christian Faith Publishing, Inc.
832 Park Avenue
Meadville, PA 16335
www.christianfaithpublishing.com

Printed in the United States of America

Contents

Introduction

This was not my intent. Neither was this my idea. At my six-tieth birthday, just after my stem cell transplant, my sister gave me an album that was a pictorial remembrance of my journey with leukemia. It had been a long two-year journey that was in parts forgotten and for many others parts that I desired to forget. She then asked me, "When are you going to write the book?" It was an idea that several had mentioned to me, but I had not taken seri-ously. In many ways, my experience was unusual. But in many oth-ers, it was routine. Perhaps my sharing could be an encouragement to individuals and families battling leukemia. Perhaps my strong faith foundation would be encouraging to those struggling with life's assaulting blows. Whatever the reason you might have chosen to read my writings, I hope what has occurred in my life may be used to help benefit yours in some way. So walk with me through this journey marked by heartache, fear, pain, spiritual confusion, faith's hope, and so many more emotions. Allow my experience to do what I under-stood God was intending it to do—to be used by Him to honor His Name and encourage His people. I am not a victim. Neither am I an object of God's cruel punishment. I am instead a follower of His, who committed myself to be used by Him in whatever way He chose. Little did I ever dream that leukemia would be His pathway for me. The album begins with the following quote from the Bible.

"Then know this, you and all the people of Israel: It is by the name of Jesus Christ of Nazareth, whom you crucified but whom God raised from the dead, that this man stands before you healed" (Acts 4:10, NIV).

And for me, there is no doubt about it!

Prepared for the Journey

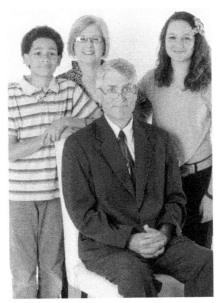

Family 2013

I lay on the emergency room bed quiet and still trying to regain my equilibrium. My mind raced through the previous two weeks and the reason for my being there. Two weeks ago, it was only a sore throat and difficulty swallowing. The nurse practitioner thought it was a severe case of tonsillitis and prescribed antibiotics, which seem to have worked, at least until the prescription ran out. The very next day, I could feel the swelling in my throat returning, so off to the doctor we went. He took note of a few additional symptoms and wanted to run a blood test. He mentioned the possibility of a more serious problem but wasn't convinced we needed to be concerned yet. Two days later, I was sitting lifelessly in my front room when my wife came in the back door. She had her cell phone in her hand and said, "The doctor wants to talk with us." The warning bells began to sound as I knew it was never good to get a call from your physician. "Earl," he said, "I don't like to talk over the phone, but this is urgent. You have tested positive for leukemia. I want you to go straight to the Medical University of South Carolina (MUSC) and do not delay. I have talked with them and they will be waiting for you." Shock was setting in. We told my sisters and began making preparation for our two children. It was already 3:00 p.m., and we had no thought of being able to return that night. My oldest sister agreed to drive my wife and me to MUSC, a three-hour trip, so we left about one hour later.

I arrived to find that they were indeed expecting me and awaiting my arrival. They quickly ushered me into an examination room and began drawing blood for their own test. Within an hour, a young doctor returned and stood at the foot of my bed. He had introduced himself earlier and let me know he was part of the cancer team. He gave me the results. "Mr. Spivey, you are testing positive for leukemia, and we will be moving you up to the cancer floor very shortly." And with that, the reality of what was happening rolled over me like a tidal wave.

That night proved to be a sleepless night of spiritual wrestling. As I soon settled into my room, the flurry of attention calmed by midnight, and I now had time to dig for the roots of my faith in search of a secure hold.

As I held my Bible and thumbed through the pages, I kept returning to one place—Gethsemane. I struggled to find some other place where God's peace could calm my fears and swirling emotions. But I couldn't get away from the garden of struggle. I found myself sensing the presence of Christ Himself as we wept and cried to the Father in search of some other way. I felt led to the suffering servant passage in Isaiah. I slowly read it seeking to be sensitive to God's message to me. It came in Isaiah 53:11. "After the suffering of his soul, he will see the light of life and be satisfied; by his knowledge my righteous servant will justify many, and he will bear their iniquities" (NIV).

And then came the "peace that passes all understanding." It was clear. I was not being punished by an angry God. I was not the victim of circumstances beyond my control. Mine was not the sad misfortune of a damaged genetic family heritage. I was chosen by God. Chosen for a path that would be marked by pain and suffering. Chosen in love to be an instrument of His work. Chosen to represent the unseen God to a world denying His existence.

"But God," I cried out, "how can I bear such a weight? How can I be used of you in such an experience?"

"I have prepared you," His answer came, "and I will enable you."

And in the words of Isaiah himself, I responded, "Here am I LORD send me." Now the battle was over. The troubled waters stilled. The anxious spirit was at peace and calm once more. For the rest of the night, I allowed God to show me the preparations He had done in making me ready for this assignment.

As a young Christian, I had made a commitment to God to be Christ's disciple. I was compelled by the Scriptures that Christ's intent for every believer is to become His follower, His student. I sought to live under the authority and control of Christ. God's reminder was that I had agreed to be used at His discretion having given myself to Him.

I was His and there was no turning back. If leukemia was the chosen path, then that was where I would choose to follow. Then God walked me back in time to see several crosses placed upon me that prepared me for this cross of leukemia. One was a cross of self-denial. In my young adult years, I, like so many others, gravitated to personal dreams and wishes. There were the dreams of marital life, personal enjoyments, achievements, and more. The conflict came as to whether I would seek my dreams or God's choices. For many years, the struggle raged. By nature, I am a headstrong, self-motivated person. So I spent many years searching for a way to lead—manipulate would be a better word—my wife into being the partner, housekeeper, and helper that I desired. Slowly, my domineering ways gave way to God's greater plan, and I came to love her for who she is and not the person I want her to be.

I enjoyed hard work and the pleasure of achievement it brought. Right out of seminary, we purchased an old house at my first pastorate, and I spent many hours working to remodel it. Much time and effort was spent in repairing and improving the structure without ever asking whether this was where I needed to be investing my energy. I was a bi-vocational pastor and worked as an appliance repairman. I was gifted with a mechanical thinking mind and loved working on things. Ten or more hours a day, I would work the service calls and other jobs around the shop. For six months, I owned the shop while the owner tried another opportunity and then returned. On top of that, I would come home to work on Bible studies and sermons. I remember a number of occasions when I dreamed of ways to make money while not working so hard. The reason was pastoring was not such a prosperous profession. Many pastors lived on the minimum and I wanted more. The question was how to minister and yet make more money than a minister's salary provided. Through Bible study and a tenacious faith, I came to have peace with accepting what was provided and learned the apostle Paul's secret of being content in every circumstance.

As I lay in my hospital room and reviewed the early years of my adult life, I could see how God had slowly molded me to accept what He gave and to be content to live obediently to Him. Over time, my will slowly was molded to His way, and I denied my selfish wants for God's assignments and entrustments.

Another cross was shown to me, the cross of self-sacrifice. It came in the form of adoption. Not every cross is marked by pain and lack of desire. This one was welcomed, even invited, but one that came at great cost all the same. My wife and I were forty-five years old and childless. It wasn't planned but just never happened. We had looked into adoption once, but it just didn't work out. We went the infertility route until the cost was too high. So we agreed that if God opened the door, we would walk through it. But if not, we would learn to be content as we were. For me, that led to many self-enjoyments and freedoms that come from not having children. I could enjoy a golf outing once a week. My extra cash could be invested in golfing, and my day off gave me time to play. I began fishing, which I enjoyed. We purchased an old boat and used our extra cash to fix it up and traded golfing for fishing. I had the freedom to work late and go in to work early. My workdays were long, and I liked it that way.

We had freedom to go out to eat regularly and time to be involved in many different activities.

Then early one morning, a phone call changed it all. The voice on the phone said, "Lauretta, we have a young lady about to give birth, and she doesn't want to keep the baby. We wanted to give you first chance before we called Social Services." Two days later, we brought home a beautiful baby girl.

Almost one year later, we got another call. This time, it is a handsome baby boy. As we adjusted to parenthood, I took seriously my spiritual obligation to father these two children. As I prayed and searched within, it was clear that to invest the love and time in my children, personal enjoyments and freedoms would have to be sacrificed. No more early-to-work and late-to-home days. No more Saturdays on the water and evenings working on a boat. No more eating out except for special occasions. Now was the time to invest in the lives of my children and share the parenting responsibilities of becoming a family.

"See," God seemed to be saying, "I prepared you to give of yourself for the good of another. In this journey, you are ready to put your self-interests aside and allow me to use you."

As the night wore on and my sleepless eyes remained wide open, the conversation continued. I saw another cross—the cross of submission. I had recently resigned from a church that I had pastored for twenty years. It had been a difficult and turbulent ride. I believed and felt various affirmations that my role was to lead the church into becoming a more modern and socially inviting congregation to its changing community. For over twelve years, we struggled with changes to the organization, church practices, and future plans. And after all that time of struggle and strife, we were almost equally divided over the direction the church should take. Unwilling to be cold and stern, I threw myself into prayer seeking godly wisdom for the situation. After a year of weekly prayer times, I felt that changing the congregation would require nothing less than a bloody revolution, and I was not going to be such a revolutionary. The church is Christ's body, and I, as its shepherd, was to nurture it and not destroy it. I didn't have a command from God to split the congregation and forcefully impose a new church. I did, however, have a biblical mandate to nurture the faith community and lead them to live under the governance of their Head, Jesus Christ.

So after many years of effort, planning, and dreaming, I chose to lay it all aside and committed myself to being the shepherd and no longer the leader of a new direction. If a new direction was taken, it would be Christ that instigated it. I was not going to heaven with a church split on my record.

"See," I could hear the Lord saying, "I was able to make you submissive to me even though it would come at great disappointment."

Now here I was in a hospital bed looking at a fearful and lengthy major illness taking another step into submissiveness. I was left to trust God with the future, as if I had any control anyway. So many dreams and future anticipations seemed to be vanishing as my awareness of what this illness would involve grew. And yet there was the peace that God was in control, and my submission was the best place for me to be.

And yet another cross came to mind. This cross was to teach me loving compassion. That was my mother's strength. She was a soft, welcoming, accepting, and compassionate person. Though I witnessed it time and time again, my strength was more like my father's—strong, determined, calculating, and honest.

I and my four sisters sat at the dining room table. My mother and father had just left the Thanksgiving meal to return to their home, and we all knew time had come to talk care giving.

A couple of years earlier, my mother was diagnosed with dementia. She had progressively grown worse, but my father had been able to provide the care she needed. Now she was experiencing physical symptoms of the disease, and her care was becoming more demanding. We had begun to notice some curious and disturbing traits in my father's behavior as well. He was a very private person so he went to the doctor alone and always returned with a glowing report. It was when my mother had to be hospitalized for a few days that we ran into my father's doctor. What he told us was not so glowing.

"Your father has dementia, too," he told us. "I would place him about a year or so behind your mother."

It was now clear that the time had come for the children to start caring for the parents. The difficulty was while Mom would go with the flow, my father would fight the tide until it went back out again. My four sisters looked at me, and we all knew that only one of us could handle the strong-willed, domineering father, his strong-willed son. The girls were more suited to care for our mother.

After several days of soul searching and Scripture reviewing, I concluded that my responsibility was to care for my parents, and hiding behind being a pastor would not be pleasing to God. So I shared my decision with my congregation, and they kindly allowed me to continue pastoring and move thirteen miles away to be closer to my parents.

I now threw myself into building a house on the family farm just behind my parent's home. After a year of construction, we moved in. It was a great comfort to my parents for us to be close and a comfort for my sisters as well. Now I began a new routine of stopping in on my way to the office each morning and again as I returned each afternoon. I was able to keep a close eye on what was happening and inform my sisters of any help needed. I was also better able to evaluate their living conditions and enable my sisters and me to respond as necessary.

And so it went for the next couple of years until my mother passed away. She had become bedridden, and I was having to spend more time helping Daddy care for her. His physical health was crumbling, and his efforts to assist my mother often proved less than what was needed.

Now, my attention was focused solely upon my father. The routine stayed the same except time spent with him after work became longer and longer. We spent hours in conversation, and I watched as his thinking and motor skills deteriorated. His strength and determination enabled him to fight dementia as he had battled the many obstacles of life. Yet, this one would eventually overpower him. For the next few years, compassion was the agenda set before me. From doctor visits to personal care, feeding to helping bathe, being present while time passes to doing what he could no longer do for himself, God was teaching me compassion.

My father and I had never been very close. We were too much like one another. We both were strong-willed and determined. We both liked things our own way and didn't give in very easily. We had mutual activities that would bring us together, but they were usually cooperative ventures for a common purpose. The teenage years made it clear that the personality we shared demanded mutual respect and room to allow for independence. Each was going to be his own man, and neither was going to dominate the other.

So it was my journey of faith that led me to honor, respect, submit, and love my father. It was what the Bible taught, and I had no choice but to apply it. Over the adult years, my appreciation for my father increased, and my efforts to show affection and respect increased. Still, there was a huge chasm that divided us, and we were two men living separate lives.

I had never pictured myself as a caregiver to my mother or father. My natural drive was to move toward my objectives and intentions disregarding other distractions. I was not, by nature, the warm and fuzzy type. Yet, my faith was changing me. I was confronted with the importance and command to love others, not use or drive them. I was finding many places in life where I had to rearrange my plans to give consideration to someone else. God was changing a tough, independent taskmaster into a person who was becoming sensitive and caring about others. Now came the ultimate test.

As I sat for endless hours listening to my father recount his past, I began to discover a father I never knew. His depth and deep feelings had been hidden by his absence due to work and other interests and by his "keep to himself" way of life. Now the curtain was parted, and I could see his fears, concerns, intended desires, and reasons for the many decisions I had only seen from the outside. I was discovering my father as a person, and compassion arose in me.

I found it most interesting that while I lay in the emergency room waiting for the doctor to tell me what my condition was, I had one overwhelming sensation. It was the presence of my father. He had died over a year before, and I often thanked God that he and my mother didn't have to live through my journey with leukemia. As I lay there lifeless and fearful, it was his presence that was powerfully felt. Not my mother's, but the father from whom I had always felt so distanced. The father with whom I had walked through the most difficult years of his life was now there beside me. It wasn't until the diagnosis was confirmed, and I was taken to my room on the cancer floor that I no longer felt his presence beside me. "See," I felt as if God were saying, "I molded you to live with compassion. Now you can, with compassion, take this journey."

And as the sun neared the horizon, there was one more cross revealed to me. It was the cross of trusting. Just six months earlier, I had taken one of the most daring steps of my life. Believing God wanted me to use some inherited property to start a ministry to single mothers, I resigned as pastor and gave myself fully to the cause. I was only fifty-six so I was too young to retire. I didn't have any other jobs awaiting. It was a bold leap of faith. A far greater leap than I imagined.

Over the years, I felt challenged in my faith to trust God with various matters and not set in action my own plan for taking care of them. Issues with raising the children became areas of trust building. Pastoring matters and personal matters became areas where I felt God wanted to work rather than wanting me to work for God. My natural personality was to devise a solution to a problem and then work it until the problem was solved. But God seemed to be guiding me in discovering how He can solve the problem and be recognized rather than my human effort. So praying and watching became a new part of my spiritual journey.

My wife is a nurse and had been working part-time since the children came. Her work was becoming irregular and sparse. We didn't have a lot of debt so the income demand wasn't great. But bills needed to be paid and without a regular income, they wouldn't be paid. That is unless God opened doors and created a cash inflow by some other means.

So, with a confirmation of trusting and depending upon God, I released the regular income and set to work on the ministry. After a couple of months, the income wasn't improving so I pulled some money from a small retirement account to carry us through the next several months. I continued to work at this ministry while praying for opportunities to speak when pastors were away or for special services. I began doing appliance repair on the side to make a little money as well. But still, no financial relief was seen.

Losing a regular income was only part of the leap of faith. The other was health insurance. My health insurance had always been one of the benefits given me as a pastor. Now that I wasn't pastoring, the cost of health insurance for my family was unthinkable. So I prayed for God's protection until we could afford the cost of insurance. For the first six months, all had gone well. But the cross of trusting was about to get much heavier and the faith to carry it much more difficult.

Here I was in a hospital where I had visited church members many times. This time, I was the one in the bed. I was about to go through major, expensive medical treatments. I was trapped in a small room with all the attention that no one wanted, and I was uninsured. As the sun rose in my room's window, all I could say was, "Lord, I'm in too deep to help myself. I'm resting in you. Lord, have mercy on my soul."

I held my Bible tightly and read Isaiah 53:11 over and over. I prayed a prayer of submission. I knew that what was about to take place for me was a cross of suffering and pain. But the results, like that of Christ Himself, would be used to affect the lives of many for God's honor and praise. And out of the garden I came, cross upon my shoulder, as the nurse entered to start the difficult journey before me.

The Road Back Home

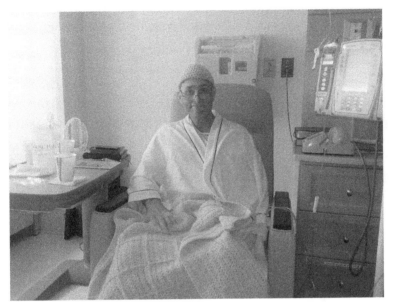

Hairless & Weak

My diagnosis was acute myeloid leukemia. It is a genetic mutation in which the white blood cells multiply at an accelerated rate. They can multiply so rapidly that the blood system is overwhelmed by them. As in my case, the white blood cells are immature and thus have no benefit in the battle against invaders. They just take up space and clog up the pathways. When that occurs, the lack of space for red blood cells leads to death. And it doesn't take long. The normal white blood cell count is between 4,500 and 10,000. When my family doctor got the results of my blood test, my white blood cell count was 70,000 and rising, and that test result was over twenty-four hours old. When I reached MUSC, my count had risen to over 90,000. The mark at which fatality usually occurs is 100,000. A few days later, the doctor talked with my wife outside my room. He said, "Mrs. Spivey, you can be thankful you got Mr. Spivey here when you did. His white blood cell count had risen to over ninety thousand and if it had gone above a hundred thousand, there would have been little we could have done." He then said, "If you had been a few hours later, we wouldn't have been able to do much for him." That was the beginning of many "it just so happened" experiences that confirmed God's hand was upon me through this journey.

They started several medications to help ease my condition. At first, I responded well, and the white blood count even dropped to below 50,000. I was starting to eat and felt the easing of the swelling in my throat. But one day is no prediction of the next, and two days after being admitted, my wife wrote the following on the CaringBridge website set up for those wanting to keep track of my condition.

> Earl J slept some. WBC back up to 90,000. Lungs congested. Did a chest X-ray, gave him prednisone and Lasix. I went to the hotel room with Mom and family last night, Elliott spent the night with his dad. Also started some new medications to work on the elevated blood counts. Earl J is not feeling well again and this with the new information is frustrating. But the Lord is with us, and we know He is walking the path by our side and carrying us when needed.

It was going to be an up and down journey filled with unexpected turns, twists, and pitfalls. The initial word was that I would only be in the hospital in two to three weeks. Now it had changed to four to six weeks. It all seemed to be getting worse quickly, but the peace of my first night held me secure.

The next day, a bone marrow biopsy was done. This was the only way to go straight to the birthing place for blood cells and see which of several causes created my leukemia. They gave me some Ativan to make me calm, as I was anxious about just what the procedure would involve. Local anesthesia was used to numb an area on my upper hip where a sizeable needle would be inserted through the hipbone and into the marrow. The doctor would use a combination of pressure and twisting motion to drill a hole in the bone and then insert the needle that would extract the marrow. I, though groggy from the medication, was greatly relieved that little pain was felt, and the procedure was more uncomfortable than painful. After this biopsy, I would no longer take a sedative but only the local anesthetic, which was enough to mask the pain. I was to have several more in the hospital and then once taking the experimental drug would have one every eight weeks or so for over a year. Sometimes in the clinic, a medical drill was used instead of the manual pressure, but neither caused much pain.

Now the preparations began. It was necessary for the nurses to have a quick and reliable access into my blood system to draw blood and inject the many medications I would need. Since I was uninsured, the lesser expensive PICC line was chosen. The PICC line was made of three external connectors that led directly into the main veins in my upper arm. It would be the direct line into my blood stream for the chemotherapy and many other medications used. I was taken to the operating room and given local numbing to the arm, while the line was inserted and then stitched to my skin to secure it. A few X-rays were taken during the procedure to insure the line was in its proper place. Now no more sticking with needles, well almost.

Once I had taken the chemotherapy, my immune system would get low, and any temperature above normal was taken seriously. When one occurred, they would immediately check for any bacterial infection. To do so, they would bypass the PICC line to get my blood sample because the external connections could be contaminated. Other than that, all my IVs would be done through the PICC line.

Once the PICC line was in, the nurses started IV lines. First was just fluid to rehydrate my system that was badly dehydrated. They added antibiotics and other little bags of which I cannot recall their contents. It would be almost eight weeks before I could experience life without being tied to lines and an IV pump machine. Any time you move, you have to adjust your lines. Even in bed at night, the lines had to be treated carefully and movement restricted so as not to damage the access site. But before long, that too became normal—a new normal.

With the line working properly and my immediate medical dangers resolved, it was time for the chemotherapy. I was not blind to the effects of chemotherapy, but I also knew that differing types of chemo have differing effects. The doctors talked with my wife and me, and we decided to let the computer decide which type we would take.

The Medical University of South Carolina (MUSC) is a teaching hospital. They are teaching future doctors and working to advance medical practices by testing new procedures and variations of existing procedures. Although my wife was a nurse, to determine if one of several types of chemo was best required more understanding than either of us had. So we agreed to participate in one of their studies evaluating the differences various chemotherapies had. All were proven to be effective, but some were believed to be more effective than others. Only testing would provide the evidence doctors needed for future treatments. If you participated, they would use the computer to randomly choose one of several treatment methods. We signed the papers and waited for our lot to be cast. It was an old standard treatment proven by the past to effectively destroy the mass of white blood cells.

I was to get a mixture of two chemotherapy drugs. One was what we referred to as one of the Rubison sisters. It was daunorubicin, which we pronounced as Donna Rubison. She had a sister Ida, idarubicin. This was another cancer treatment, but I was selected to go with Donna. She would have all the familiar side effects. I would battle nausea, eventually lose my hair, and possibly deal with some other unpleasant conditions. But my choices were slim.

When my wife returned from being back home several days with our children, she wrote this post on CaringBridge.

> I am back with Earl J. Rough morning for me emotionally. Prayer, encouraging words pulled

me through the valley. Earl J's face was flushed when I arrived, an effect of the drugs. When I asked him how he was doing, he said, "I'm just letting the waves roll over me." Christine and Elliott returned to school this morning. Earl J's sister (Patricia) will bring them down after school on Friday. Earl J was started on two chemotherapy drugs yesterday evening. He in getting the 7+3 regimen. The 3 in the equation is daunorubicin, he receives it once a day for 3 days. The 7 is cytarabine, which will infuse 24 hours a day for 7 days. The doctors state the worst of the side effects will most likely hit on days 4–6. That will be this weekend and might not be a good time for visits. Hugs and kisses are to be limited. Earl J requested his flute and hymnal, CD player, and CDs. He is playing the flute now, which will be good for his lungs. "Why art thou cast down, O my soul? And why art thou disquieted within me? Hope in God: for I shall yet praise Him, who is the health of my countenance, and my God." (Ps. 43:5)

The treatment started uneventfully, just the constant dripping of chemo into my blood stream along with fluids. I was feeling better now that the condition in my throat had improved, and I was able to eat and regain some strength. Though weak, I was getting better for the moment. I had to use trial and error methods on the hospital food. I had a menu from which I could choose. But my expectations were not always the reality that greeted me once I removed the plate cover. So I learned the foods that I could eat and tried to keep a balanced diet as I knew I would need all the strength I could build.

When one bag of fluid or chemo ran out, another was quickly replacing it. And once a day came the changeup with an injection of daunorubicin. Other than that, that was the daily routine of taking my vitals—oxygen level, blood pressure, temperature, and heart rate.

Each day, your weight was taken. It usually occurred at four in the morning. Sometimes, it happened at midnight, but four was the designated hour. The vitals were taken every four hours.

They wanted to keep a close eye on my heart so a telemonitor was given to me. It was a weighty mass that hung around my neck with several leads to my chest and abdomen. It was worn 24/7 and only took a few minutes to detest. Bulky and dangling from your neck, always in an uncomfortable position, you found it hard to grow accustomed to its presence. Whether sitting in the foldout chair, lying in bed, or just moving about the weighty necklace seemed to be in an annoying place.

As the days began to count up, so was my strength counting down. I had entered the hospital a strong and healthy fifty-eight-year-old though weakened from the sickness. I was encouraged to walk the hall and get as much exercise as I could. So I did but felt myself winding down like a weakening battery. After just a few days of chemotherapy, my energy was going fast. The side effects were setting in and nausea was a constant hindrance. Here is what my wife wrote just one week into the journey.

> We are getting through some of the shock. There is still so much to process. Earl J and I feel God's love and very prevalent presence. He is our Rock and Strength. Overall, it has been a good day. Earl J ate breakfast and lunch with minimal nausea. Felt woozy and queasy a few times moving around. And he walked some. This morning, his WBC was 2,000 and platelets 8,000. He did get platelets around lunchtime. The weakness continues and gradually increases.

I could feel the strength of my independence for fifty-eight years slipping away. I knew that I was heading into a time when others would increasingly care for me as I would be unable to care for myself. The daily walks down the hallways became more and more an effort. The determination to continue them demanded more and more inner strength. It would have been so easy to give in and give up. But I had a cross to carry, and quitting was not an option.

As mentioned earlier, I grew up with a determined personality. I often thought of myself as a mule in spirit. I was just old enough to remember my father working two mules on the farm where I lived. I was very young, and it wasn't long before they were replaced with tractors. But mules had a more determined spirit than horses. The mule would pull the plow and work for the farmer consistently, persistently, and long past the time when a horse would quit. I was a hard worker and often found my mule-natured spirit my salvation. Many of my successes were due to my continuous determination more than my intelligence or wisdom. And now I faced the ultimate test. To walk the hallway, go to the bathroom, or just get up and move about in the room seemed to require a major effort. Eating was a necessary but no longer enjoyable part of life. First, it was work. Second, it seemed to always be laced with nausea. Third, my tastes were changing.

It didn't take long for the side effects to start. The growing nausea became a twenty-four-hour battle. The doctors and nursing staff were very good and generous about it. They wanted me to eat as much as I could and keep my strength up as long as possible. They knew what was ahead and the importance of my being strong with as much momentum as I could muster. So they encouraged me to not wait until I felt like I was going to throw up. Instead I was to attack the nausea early on and keep it down. I was given a list of medications to use against it and could use them almost at will. Zofran, Phenergan, Compazine, and even Ativan were all at my disposal.

I didn't want to take medications and had never had to take any for ailments. So I evaluated the side effects of each and used the lesser of the perceived evils. That was a good strategy, I thought, so Zofran was the choice every six hours. It was then that I discovered one little warning I had not noticed.

My wife had battled migraine headaches for years. I had often seen that look on her face that told of intense pain. I watched her retreat into isolation with pillow over the head and the room as dark as possible. I never knew what she experienced and couldn't empathize with her, only seldom having a minor headache. But that was about to change.

One of the side effects of Zofran can be migraine headaches. Thinking the side effects would be minimal, I indulged myself. After a short time, I began to experience intense pain in my head. I also noticed that the light was intense and painfully bright. I shared what was happening with the nurses and doctors, and they confirmed that I had just discovered the migraine headache. So I began to alternate Phenergan with the Zofran and in a day of two, the migraine left. That has made me much more sympathetic toward my wife during her migraine moments. I often remember what my brother-in-law shared after that. He, too, had battled migraines most all his life. When they grew real intense, he would go to a physician for some relief. He said, "I could always tell when the doctor knew the pain I was experiencing. He would come into the room, speak softly, and turn the lights off." It became one of many experiences that would heighten my compassion for others by understanding their pain and discomfort.

But if the nausea wasn't enough, my mouth was undergoing a most unwanted transformation. Years before, I had undergone surgery to relieve some of the effects of childhood polio. Tendons in the toes of my right foot were severed to relieve their drawing up, hammer toe effect. A tendon on the inside of my ankle was split and then attached to the outside of my foot to give me more support while walking and running. The pain medications following the surgery left me nauseated much of the time. The one thing I could still eat without being sick was Hershey's Kisses. So I ate a lot of them and often during sick times would rely on them to help me through. My wife had prepared for the occasion, and I had a good supply on hand. But I began to notice a strange taste when letting one slowly dissolve—the only way to eat one—in my mouth. A bitterness was sensed. I ate a few more and to my great horror discovered that the candy was fine. It was my taste that was changing.

Food ordered became, for the most part, tasteless. What once was an enjoyable mouth full of flavor was now a mouth full of flavorless, multitextured material. The once inviting aroma of a cooked meal was now a stench you were barely able to endure to take a few bites of the cuisine.

And on top of all that was the change of texture and mouth sensation. I had always enjoyed a cheeseburger. So when my sister was on her way to see me, she called me to see if I wanted anything. "A cheeseburger," I told her with great anticipation. *Surely*, I thought, *food outside the hospital would not be so bad.* Soon she arrived with cheeseburger in hand. With eager anticipation of what one tasted like only a week or so earlier, I pulled back the wrapper and sank my teeth into the seed-covered bun, hot melted cheese, and juicy hamburger patty and almost spit it out. It was tasteless. The more I chewed it, the more like Styrofoam it felt. My salivary glands were no longer producing the needed fluids to moisten and bring out the flavors of the food. Instead, there was the dry, tasteless mass being pulverized by my teeth and passed down my throat under great resistance. And that would be the new norm for many weeks. How could I maintain any strength like this?

Just a week into however long this hospital stay was going to last, I was starting to form new routines. I was confined to the room other than the periodic walks taken on this specialized floor. I had broken the TV habit some many years earlier. It came about as I noticed that I was watching TV because I just didn't want to do anything else. There were many more beneficial things to be doing, but TV gave me the opportunity to do something without doing anything. Also, I found myself more aware of the ideas and concepts being presented through the various programming that spiritually I opposed. Not wanting my mind filled with more things that contradicted my belief than social interactions already created, I decided to break the habit. At first, it was awkward and uncomfortable. But soon, it proved to be an experience freeing me to invest in other more meaningful and beneficial experiences.

So as Lauretta mentioned in the preceding post, I asked for my recorder, Bible, and CDs. Bible reading had become an important part of my day. It was an early morning moment that allowed me to collect my thoughts and focus them on my spiritual identity each day. It also was a special time to discover the many insights, directives, and corrections the Scriptures can make in our living. As I customarily awoke about five thirty or six o'clock each morning, I arranged my time with God within my hospital routine. Usually, about 6:00 a.m., the nurse would enter with a medication I needed to take in the early morning. I found that once the medication was taken, the nurse would not return till seven fifteen or seven thirty when the shift changed and the new nurse would be introduced to me. After the nurse left at 6:00 a.m., I had over an hour of uninterrupted time. So for the first few weeks, I would take my Bible in hand and continue the familiar and comforting routine of reading the Bible first thing in the day.

Prayer had become an important practice for me as well. It had become a mixture of daily worship and surrender. I believe Jesus Christ to be Lord of all, and I had committed myself to be one of His followers. Prayer became one of the essential spiritual disciplines in my living. I had learned that too often, we pray with a half-hearted attitude. We share a few thoughts and requests with God and only then do so while moving through our busy activities. Fellowship with God takes time, just as a conversation with a dear friend requires our time and attention. I had therefore returned to the age-old practice of carving out time and kneeling when I prayed. It caused me to remember the amazing God before whom I came and also my need to approach Him in humbleness. It also, due to the unnatural position, helped me keep focused and alert rather than falling back asleep in bed or an easy chair. Not every morning availed itself to times of prayer, but many times until my strength grew very weak, I would make my way over to the foldout chair and kneel for my morning prayers. Only once or twice was I interrupted, but even then, it was a witness of my faith.

The recorder was one of the simplest musical instruments to play. It is often used for beginning music students. Years earlier, I was moved by hearing one on a worship CD and decided to put down my guitar and pick up the recorder. I participated in the church instrumental group with my guitar so now I added the recorder. Its soft sound and small size made it very convenient for taking it places. I was not an accomplished player by any means, but I enjoyed playing it and had always loved the hymns of my faith. On many days, I could use up several hours of the long hospital day just playing hymn after hymn on the recorder. On many occasions, I found myself having to stop and just take in the powerful message the old hymns shared. I also found an unexpected advantage. A number of the nurses would come by my room and encourage me to keep playing the hymns. They recalled the songs, and many still sung them. Though my door was closed, the soft sound was flowing down the hallway, and hearts were being refreshed by the sound of the ancient musical messages of faith.

My CDs were a collection of hymns, contemporary and classical music. As I passed the hours when my concentration was low or I just wanted to sit quietly, I would play a CD and relax. They proved to be a great comfort in passing the time that seemed to move so slowly in the hospital. I often lay in bed looking at the clock on the wall wondering if it had been slowed down by some adjustment. Time passed slowly and the music did much to encourage my spirit as the environment was slowly taking its toll.

I was now finishing the chemo treatment. The weight of its effect was building. My energy was going fast and my "want to" was fading quickly as well. Every morning about 4:00 a.m., a blood sample would be drawn so tests could be made and the results ready for the doctor when rounds were made. My tests revealed the quick deterioration of my blood system. The destructive force of the chemo was destroying my blood cells as well as my marrow. As a result, my platelet count was dropping, and bags of platelets were hung on the IV pole to be slowly pumped into my system. Also, pint after pint of blood was given to keep my organs functioning and alive. No longer was my bone marrow producing the red blood cells, white blood cells, and platelets. As my system was destroyed, all needed blood components would have to be added from outside my body. One of the humbling experiences of my treatment was looking at the bags of platelets or red blood cells and wondering who provided life for me. Without them, I would die quickly. But due to those who donated blood, I would be kept alive with greater hopes for tomorrow.

Just over a week into the treatment, the order was given. "Visitation is to be restricted to family and only those not sick or have been around those who are sick. Visitors are to wear surgical masks to prevent the passing of viruses and bacteria." Those staying with me were freed from the constant wearing of the mask. However, all precautions were to be taken to prevent my contact with any virus, infectious illness, or bacteria. The reason was my immune system. With the destruction of my blood system came the removing of my immune system. No more production of white blood cells, and they were the one blood component that could not be received from another person. The doctors could give antiviruses, antifungal meds, and antibacterial drugs, but I was now helpless to fight against even the simplest invader to my body. So only two options were available. First, prevent any infection before it occurred. Second, respond to any infection with a massive medical assault. It would take weeks following the chemo treatment, even months, before my immune system would return. Now I had entered the most critical time of the treatment, the most dangerous place, the time when it was the easiest to catch a virus or bacterial infection and die before the assault could counteract it.

As you can imagine, the hospital took this seriously. Masks were everywhere, latex gloves were always worn, and alcohol swabs were used till the room smelled like a brewery. And if you forgot and walked into the hallway without a mask, a compassionate sharp chastisement was soon upon you. Above my bed was a constant blowing of air. The ventilation system was especially designed for this condition. The air never stopped flowing, and it passed through a series of anti-everything filters. The rooms were even designed so that when the door was opened, the inside air pushed out instead of the hallway air coming in. I would amuse myself by watching the little green ball that looked like a ping-pong ball flip back and forth in the clear tube just above the door. It let the nurses know that the air pressure conditions were as desired in the room.

At the two-week mark of my hospital stay, I learned of another anti-infectious method. I was lying in my bed in the early evening when several nurses and techs, those taking my vitals, entered the room. They began collecting my things and said, "Mr. Spivey, you get another room tonight." *But I don't want another room*, I thought. They then explained that to fight against the threat of infection, each patient was moved every two weeks, and the room was cleaned from top to bottom. So out I went with my belongings being carried behind me. I was quickly settled into another room on the same floor and allowed to return to my evening rest. The old room was then scrubbed, dusted, sanitized inch by inch, and made ready for another patient.

The chemo was past, but its effects grew. The doctors said that the chemo would peak in its effects in about twenty-one days. A biopsy could be done on day 14 to measure the effectiveness of the chemo. So another biopsy would be done shortly. Days passed slowly, but day 14 finally arrived. Three weeks in the hospital. Weak and fighting to get up and walk, I clung to the new normal; the daily routines that gave me some structure and way to live each day.

By now, I had gone from 175 pounds to 165. Eating was unpleasant, and the desire for food just wasn't there. I was thankful that the side effects I was experiencing didn't include mouth sores and other more painful conditions. As it was, my side effects were considered mild and for that, I was thankful.

Blood and platelets were a regular part of my diet. It seemed to me that Donna, daunorubicin, was doing her part pretty well. We were all hopeful that one time through would be enough. But we knew that the final word would come from the biopsy, and we held our breath and prayed.

It took a couple of days to get the results and the report was, "Cancer cells still present in the marrow." It was a great disappointment to everyone. For me, it was one of my faith-testing times. The doctor explained that a second round of chemo would be necessary. The same combination, but this time, the strength would be less as the cancer was not as advanced. Even with that, I could anticipate the present side effects to remain throughout the second treatment. After fourteen days, another biopsy would be performed, and the future would be determined then.

Needless to say, much time in prayer was made. I cried out for strength to walk the pathway set now before me. The diagnosis of leukemia, confinement to the hospital, chemo treatment and side effects were a cross heavy enough, I thought. And now, I must enter it again. I'm weak, tired, and struggle to eat. But dread could never change reality so I regrouped and set my mind to facing another round of chemo.

Here is some of what I shared with those keeping up with my struggle by way of CaringBridge.

> Brothers and sisters, let me encourage you not to become disheartened. We have been praying for God to do a complete work with the chemotherapy and to let the side effects be less intense. God has answered our request for mild side effects, but He has chosen for a second round of chemotherapy to be given. This is not failure on our part or disregard on God's. Most often, when God denies our request, it is for a greater purpose. As Christ's servant and minister, I accept His greater purpose for my life. This second time through the chemotherapy promises to be more difficult due to my already weakened state. So now my cross becomes heavier, but with the weight comes a greater purpose.

With a new determination, I awaited the nurse's entrance with new bags and the beginning of round two of chemo treatment.

It was about this time that I noticed some changes that would alter my daily routines for the rest of my stay. I had increasing difficulty in focusing my vision while reading. I had also noticed that when I tried to watch a local televised worship service, where a friend from years before pastored, my vision was unfocused. The slightly blurry image made it difficult to watch. I also noticed that I couldn't read many of the words on the TV screen either. Along with the lack of focus, I now began to see spots that obstructed my view.

Reading was no longer possible as much of the words, or notes in the hymns, were blocked out by the spots. My doctor called for an eye examination, and the optometrist shined his little light into my eyes and looked carefully with the magnification instrument and gave the diagnosis, bleeders. The chemo had thinned my blood to the point that the blood vessels in my eyes were seeping blood into the fluid in my eyeballs. The result was obstructing spots and blurred vision. The remedy would be to give me more platelets and keep my blood from remaining so thin. The good news was that in time, they would disappear from my vision.

For the first time in my life, I could no longer read the Bible, other books or notes in the hymnal. I could see enough to move about and do the basic functions but not enough to focus on print. My strength was getting weak enough that getting down on my knees seemed unadvisable and too difficult to get back up without another's help. I remember crying out to God for some comfort as my spiritual disciplines that had long given me peace and strength were now taken from me. I remember well the peace I received. "I am holding you in my arms. Rest yourself in my care, and I will hold you through the troubles." And I wept to know God loved me so much that He would carry me when I was unable to walk myself. Time after time, I clung to this comfort.

It would be weeks before my eyes cleared enough for me to read again. But I could still listen. On many occasions, I asked those visiting me to read passages from the Bible to me. Those became special times when someone sat by my side and read for me what I could no longer read for myself. I would listen and give thanks that I was being carried through my troubles.

Three weeks turned into four weeks, and it was time for the second round of chemo. The routine familiar side effects were anticipated, but the severity was underestimated. What I thought would be a repeat of the time before proved to be far from reality.

Much of the strength with which I was able to withstand the first round was used up. Now I would face another round of chemo, though some lighter than the first, in a more weakened condition. That meant that the stress of the chemo would now be heavier, and the weaker areas of my body would begin to show the unacceptable effects.

The first area to buckle was my lungs. Difficulty breathing soon began bothering me. X-rays were taken, and fluid was found. Breathing treatments were started, and more X-rays ordered almost every day. If one day seemed better, the next was worse. This became a plaguing condition, which I took home with me. The breathing treatments were barely able to keep me off oxygen and soon, even that would fail.

The second area to buckle was my heart. I remember well the day the tech was making her routine round, with the cuff on my arm, thermometer in my mouth, and oxygen sensor on my finger while I sat in my foldout chair. "Mr. Spivey, I need for you to get in your bed."

"But I'm fine. Can't I just stay in my chair?"

"Mr. Spivey, I really need you to get in your bed."

So I did and soon learned the reason, atrial fibrillation. It is a condition of the heart when the regular beating rhythm is replaced with a spasmodic quivering of the heart. The heart rate goes sky high, and all the hospital staff are just filled with excitement. As for me, I didn't feel any different and just wanted to get out of my bed, but doctors and nurses forbid such. My mother had dealt with this condition. On a couple of occasions, she had had her heart shocked back into its regular rhythm. I had never experienced it to my knowledge until now. Told to stay in my bed and given more attention than I wanted I felt even more confined.

The daily routines were getting fewer and more unpredictable. My daily strength was fading, and I moved only the minimal amount necessary and just what I could to stay out of bed. For now, bed was my only option.

It was now almost five weeks and the end was still not in sight. The third bone marrow biopsy was done to evaluate the effectiveness of the second round of chemo. A long agonizing weekend slowly passed as we awaited the results. Finally, on Monday, the results came. "Less than five percent of blast cells remain." Our hope was for zero. But at least, we were almost rid of the leukemia cells. That was initially good enough to not anticipate a third round of chemo in the hospital, but another biopsy would be done in about a week and a half to show which cells were starting to grow back and a final decision would be made. So now, it would be at least seven weeks in the hospital.

By now, the mental struggle was setting in. I had been able to hope in going home and push back the dark weight of hospital confinement. With my weakening condition, inability to bathe myself, hardly able to go to the bathroom by myself and now word that all this would continue for another two weeks settled dark and heavy. It was more and more difficult to not be depressed. The music, encouragement of others, and "mule-natured" faith helped me grip tighter and not fall into despair. My thoughts were growing difficult to stay positive. I wasn't really sure if I would get home again. I felt the presence of danger constantly around me; and for good reason as the wheels were coming off my wagon.

My lungs were getting worse, and nothing was making them better. Now, a cough was starting and breathing even more difficult. Oxygen was the next step to enable me to get the needed oxygen to my system when I wasn't breathing large enough amounts of air to do so. *One more something else*, I thought, as they put the tub around my ears and under my nose. I lay in bed wondering if I would ever get out again.

To make matters even worse for my lungs, my atrial fibrillation was back and forth. It seemed to be more back than forth, and a close eye was monitoring it. I already had a new team of doctors from the lung department, and now I had a team from the heart department. Each day, my cancer doctors would make their round. Then the lung doctors would come by and then the heart doctors. By then, it was lunchtime, though eating wasn't of much interest for me.

Congestive heart failure was common with atrial fibrillation. If the heart was not beating properly, the blood was not circulating as it should, and the water that would normally be moved to the kidneys and removed would build up in the lungs and heart area. Just what I needed, water in my already drowning lungs. On one of my worse days, I gained twenty pounds of water. I still can't imagine where the water came from 'cause I know I never drank that much in a day. Needless to say, the injections of Lasix came quickly, and I found more strength than I thought I had to get out of bed and fill the bottle so they could measure the amount of water I excreted. I think they measured everything but your belching. Sometimes, I just sat on the toilet and said to myself, "If they want to measure it, they will just have to find it. I don't care!" And then, I flushed it with a smile.

> Yesterday (Monday) was quite a busy one for Earl J. He was still having problems with atrial fibrillation, shortness of breath, and fluid retention. This with the previous rounds of chemotherapy put stress on his heart causing the heart to work harder and tire. Heart rate increasing even higher and increased shortness of breath had them moving Earl J to ICU. Denley came on Monday morning so I left for home about noon. I was 30 minutes from the house when Denley called with the news. I went on home, cleaned up, handled a few household chores and returned to MUSC, arriving about 9:30PM. This morning (Tuesday) more of the same with heart, but the rate is lower (110–150). He is breathing better. A lot of doctors have been in and out (cardiology and oncology teams). The cardiologist told us Earl J had a small, mild non-STEMI heart attack. The cardiologists have spent the day trying to keep his heart regulated without much success. I get the feeling they have been frustrated at times. I know they are working hard, along with the nursing staff, and have done a wonderful job. We have faith in them, but our ultimate *faith* is with our Heavenly Father.

It was the bottom of the barrel, and the bottom seemed like a huge plateau. I lay in ICU and didn't really care where I was. I had little drive to work hard to get anywhere else. I was washed out, past tired, and mentally about spent. My wife was by my side all the way using all the nursing skills she had learned over the many years of her practice. She encouraged me as best she could as my spouse of thirty plus years. Doctors came and went, and the ICU nurse kept a constant watch. Slowly, my heart stabilized, and my condition was still dangerous but controllable.

I stayed only a couple of days in ICU. I remember painfully walking around the block. If I wanted to get out, I had to get up and move so I searched for the mule within my spirit and grabbed the walker and began to walk. With the heart rate down and my condition stabilized, I was allowed to return to the cancer floor as soon as a room was available.

Needless to say, I didn't walk back to my room on the cancer floor. But when they rolled my bed into the room, it was a relief to be away from the ICU's many gadgets and noises.

As the old saying goes, "It is often darkest just before dawn," and how true that is. My situation seemed the darkest and bleakest at that moment. Hear the confusion and turmoil in my wife's post on CaringBridge.

> I kind of left things hanging with the last journal. Things were changing as soon as they changed. Earl J was going into overload and so was I. Medications were changing. Cardiology was taking over his care, then he was back under oncology for about an hour before placed back under cardiology. He was moved from ICU to the hematology unit, then was to be moved to the cardiac unit and within 30 minutes, they were keeping him on hematology unit. Then he was told he would be getting chemotherapy again in 3 weeks. Too much within an hour and a half time period for him to process on top of not feeling well.

I was back on the cancer floor, but no one seemed to know what to do with me. What was my dominant problem and most critical need? My lungs, heart, or cancer, if all were critical, where should the focus be? As the dust finally settled, I stayed on the cancer floor, and the cancer doctors continued to lead the effort.

By now, my weight was down about twenty-five pounds. Though I was able to walk, it took all the energy I could squeeze and then it wasn't far. IV pole and oxygen tank in tow, I would huff and puff to stay on my feet. My need for oxygen was constant, and I knew I was getting close to giving up.

The fourth bone marrow biopsy revealed that there were still leukemia cells present in my marrow so a third round of chemo would be needed. "I can't take it again," I said to myself. "Another round of this and I'll be dead!" It was then that the dawn began to appear, and the hope of sunrise came.

> The oncology team just came in the room. Cardiology has released him to the care of oncology. They have all cardiac prescriptions ready. Oncology is going to monitor his need for oxygen today, if his saturation is below 90% he will come home with oxygen for a week, if above no oxygen. *Then he may come home this afternoon/ evening.* God is working on this, and we give Him all the praise and glory. Amen and Amen!

I was lost in the swirling waters of hope and despair. I remember telling my wife, "They are sending me home to die." Hope was almost gone, and the joy of going home was drowned in the perception that I had fallen too far. How could I ever overcome this? But there were little signs I, in my darkness, failed to see.

The side effects of the chemo were fading. Though I was weak and had several serious conditions, my ability to eat without nausea was starting to return. I was regaining my taste for certain foods, and this would increase in time. My blood system was beginning to rebuild. Red blood cells, platelets, and the white blood cells were returning. I was out of the most dangerous condition regarding my immune system. Though the leukemia wasn't gone, at least my body was coming back from all the damage.

The doctor took me into the hallway. He removed my oxygen and said let's walk. He put an oxygen sensor on my finger and watched closely. I took a few steps and breathed heavily. The numbers on the sensor dropped quickly. After a few more steps, he said, "That's enough. Let's put your oxygen on and return to your room." *Won't be going home like this*, I thought. But back in the room, he said, "We'll make you an order for oxygen, and it will be at your home when you get there." And with that, my IVs were removed, and my wife began preparing for us to leave.

I had been in the hospital for almost eight weeks. I still had congestion in my lungs, and my heart wasn't sure to just what kind of rhythm it wanted to dance. I was bony and looked like death would have been to me relief. I wasn't sure I could handle three hours in a car needed to get home. But something deep within kept saying, "If I'm gonna die, then I'm gonna die at home."

In a state of disbelief, I eased my way into a familiar car. Oxygen tank at my feet, backseat full of medical equipment, and trunk full of belongings, my wife started the car and I knew I was finally leaving MUSC. I counted the familiar landmarks along the way and slept past many more. I twisted and turned in my seat but knew if I held on, home would soon be in sight. My emotions began to break as we crossed the bridge that marked the border of the Independent Republic of Horry County. We passed through the county seat where I had pastored for twenty years and began the final thirteen miles home. The anticipation grew with each familiar landmark. A road so often traveled now led this homesick and broken-down soul back to a place called home. As we turned off the road and down the lane leading to a log house in the middle of a field where my childhood was spent, my eyes began to water and my heart gave thanks. By God's grace, I was home once more. For how long, I didn't care. I was just back home again.

With the help of others, I shuffled my way in the door and paused to take in a place I thought I might never see again. I was not in complete remission and would have to return in a week for the next treatment but for now, I was with family, and home is the best place to heal.

A Year of Waiting

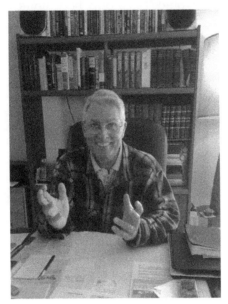

Months after Diagnosis

I came home in October of 2014, and it would not be till March of 2016 that I would reenter MUSC for the stem cell transplant. It was a time of being frustrated with the government and anxious about my medical condition. However, I soon saw it as a blessing from God. For over a year, I was given the gift of my family. I was to recover my health enough that I could ride the tractor, run a chainsaw, and do light work with the volunteers working on the ministry under development. It was more than a delay. It was a gift to be treasured. I knew that I was only home because God touched my life with many miracles. I also knew that the odds of my surviving the stem cell transplant was only about 50–60 percent. God had miraculously brought me home. I did not automatically assume He would bring me through the dangers of the transplant. So this was my time to be with family, invest in the developing ministry, and honor God for all He had done for me.

I was to avoid all crowds, but there was one crowd I longed to enter. This was the Sunday crowd of God's worshippers. For eight Sundays, I had not been able to gather with fellow believers in worship. This Sunday, I would. I had only been home a few days. I was still on oxygen, weak and unable to walk into the church. But I had a wheelchair. It belonged to my mother when dementia had limited her ability to walk. We dusted it off, and it became my mode of transportation for the next month.

Sunday brought a beautiful October morning. My wife and my two children accompanied me, surgical mask, chair, oxygen, cap on my baldhead, and all else. My wife pushed me into the sanctuary, and we took our place for the worship hour. We were in my childhood home church. Though I couldn't stand for the songs and didn't have the breath to sing, my heart rejoiced and I worshipped the One who brought me through the many recent troubles. It was more than refreshing and a recharging of my spiritual battery.

After many friendly greetings and assurances of prayer, we returned home. Of all the things I missed during my hospital stay, worship was at the top of my list. I was finally back among the crowd of worshippers, and I rejoiced to be with them again. The return home proved to be the best medicine taken so far. My wife recorded my progress as follows:

> Earl J went to morning worship the last 2 Sundays. Since coming home, it has been a long haul for him. He knew it would be a struggle but wanted to see that light at the end of the tunnel. He is seeing it this week. First by not having to sleep with his upper body propped up quite as high and sleeping through most of a night. Then He said, "I was able to stand up the whole time while brushing my teeth." Last night, he slept without having to turn the O2 up. He went to see 2 of Elliott's soccer games and plans to go Thursday

to hear Christine play the steel drums in a group
for a pep rally. He is getting stronger each day.

My strength was returning slowly but not easily. The beginning was marked by struggle. I was confined to an oxygen hose and always feeling a need for a little more. As mentioned, the standing to brush my teeth was a major effort. Moving about required patience and persistence while using a walker. But at least, I was starting to eat and that had great benefits.

The first week was a trying one. I couldn't sleep in my bed because I had to elevate my upper body to be able to breathe. I instead tried to sleep in my recliner that my wife and mother-in-law purchased just for the occasion. But sleep was hard to get. Each day, about dusk, I could feel the demand for oxygen increasing. I would turn up the concentrator a couple of notches and try to relax. For two nights, I couldn't close my eyes. I would move from one chair to the other and breathe in all the oxygen my tubes would give me. My mind would not slow down, and nothing I tried seemed to help ease my mind and allow me to sleep. Wide awake, I would spend the night going from chair to chair straining to satisfy my impulse for oxygen. I felt like the world around me was closing in, and I was about to be smothered by it.

I found this to be a deeply troubling matter for me spiritually. If God was my comfort and I trusted in His care, then why was I not able to rest in peace? Why was I so agitated and disturbed? I felt defeated. Yet there was no peace, just more anxiety.

We were to return after a few days to Hollings Cancer Center at MUSC for a doctor's visit, and my anxiety would be one of the issues discussed. I remember being taken to the waiting room. It was a normal-sized waiting room, like in most other doctor offices. It wasn't really small, but to me, it was like being shoved into a barrel. As the tech closed the door and left to let the doctor know I was there, I began to break out in a sweat. My wife looked over at me and noted my wide eyes and nervous actions. "Are you okay?" she asked. "If she (the doctor) doesn't hurry, I'm gone. This room is closing in on me."

My doctor soon came in and noticed my agitation as well. We talked about my being up at night and my anxious nature during the dark hours. She reassured me that it wasn't anything permanent or any emotional or psychological abnormality. It was part of the stress of my treatments and the physical need for oxygen. She gave me a prescription for Ativan and told me to take one before dark each night. I did and soon fell asleep in my chair. After a week or so, I was able to breathe more freely and no longer needed Ativan.

I found myself struggling to go back to the routines once so common for me. But there were no common routines anymore. To get to the table to eat required the use of a walker or wheelchair. To go to the bathroom required the assistance of my wife who became more personally involved than I desired. But with little strength, bad equilibrium, and no stamina to do anything, I was like a helpless child. To get a shower, I used the wheelchair at first and later the walker to get into the shower stall and sit on a shower chair. I was not even able to wash my legs and arms and neck. I would sit in the chair with my wife using the handheld showerhead to wet and then rinse me with tears in my eyes as I felt so helpless and so humbled at her patience and dedication.

I would flash back to just a few years earlier when it was my father in the shower chair and me with the showerhead. I had no idea what he was feeling until now. I had sought to be caring and sensitive but could now feel the personal humiliation he felt not being able to simply bathe himself. But I could also thank God to have done so, as now I felt a different love in my wife's kind actions. It was an undesired but completely willing act coming from a love that went far deeper than self's pleasure. She was fulfilling our vow, "for better or for worse…in sickness or in health." This was a "worst" time for us but love prevailed.

It was encouraging when I wanted to see my son play soccer to have others jump to help me. My wife rustled the wheelchair out of the trunk, and I would ease out of the car seat with her help to sit in it. Before she could get me settled, two or three men would be by our side ready to push me across the grassy field. And when the game was over, they would quickly be back to escort me back to the car. My weakness revealed to me people still with a kindness and readiness to help others. Society may seem busy and uncaring, but when needs are seen, there are still many compassionate souls who are willing and ready to help.

As the nighttime anxiety began to ease and my eating improved, I began to see some light. *Maybe I'm not going to die after all*, I thought. *Maybe I can regain my strength.* And I began to push toward the light of a new day when I could care for myself, return to the outdoor activities, and resume the life I abruptly left some nine weeks ago.

The joy of eating had not yet returned, but the ability to taste what I ate and not be so repulsed by the aroma was making mealtime more desirable. The relaxing of my straining on the oxygen hose enabled me to release the anxious struggle for air. And with that, the little growth in strength gave me hope of the return of independence. But that was still a long way down the road.

After a couple of weeks home, I was to return to Charleston to go through another round of chemo. Only this time, it would not require me to be in the hospital. Instead, I would be placed in a local hotel and travel back and forth to Hollings Cancer Center each day for the infusions. The arrangements were all made for us and with a renewed spirit, I returned to battle another round of chemo. This time, the chemo was a different kind and was much weaker than what was used while I was in the hospital.

My doctor had chosen a weaker chemo because, in her honesty, I was too weak to undergo another round of the same one. The weaker should be strong enough to finish the job. That would secure my suppression of leukemia's progress. Once stopped, we could then keep it under control until a transplant could be done.

So back in the car went the walker, wheelchair, supplies for the week, and my oxygen concentrator. I was amazed at how much my wife could squeeze into our compact car. We checked into the hotel, settled in for the night, and made ready for the week ahead.

I would report in each morning to have my blood tested before receiving my chemo infusion. If needed, I could also get red blood cells, platelets or whatever else my body needed. So Monday morning, we entered Hollings Cancer Center of which I became so intimately acquainted for the next two years.

43

The PICC line made me very grateful with all the drawing of blood and infusing of blood products. It was moving to sit in the waiting room or being taken to one of the rooms, in which the wall facing the hall and nurses' desk was open. Moving because you could see the many patients coming and going all suffering from cancer or a life-threatening blood condition. Many were bald, some like myself in wheelchairs, others with walkers or canes. Some seemed strong and healthy while others so frail and fragile. And one after another came in for blood test and/or infusions of chemo or blood products.

You were given a foldout chair and a pillow for comfort. You were told to bring snacks and your medications. If you were there to get an infusion, you could expect to stay from two to four hours at least. A snack or sometimes a meal would help keep your strength up and not leave you weaker when finished. I usually just had a snack and waited till I left to stop for a meal on the way back to the hotel. Sometimes, I wouldn't feel like stopping anywhere so we would get something to go or just eat what we had at the hotel.

Needless to say, it was a long tiring week. By midweek, the effects were starting to show. The familiar fatigue and nagging nausea were returning. I traded what little walking I had done earlier that week for a ride in the wheelchair. I felt the weight of sickness descending on me again but knew in just a few more days, I could go home again. Day after day, I went into the clinic, had blood drawn, and waited to get the infusion of chemo. Finally, Friday came and after a busy day of packing and getting my last infusion, we made the long trip home. It may have been dark, but the sight of home brought a renewed determination to press through this present setback.

In spite of the chemo treatment the first week in November, it was a month of slow growth. After returning from Charleston, I was weaker due to the treatment, but my breathing was slowly getting better. I could now sleep without the help of Ativan. I was feeling freer with my breathing and even began turning the oxygen down a notch or two. With the using of Bumex to remove excess water from my system, I was able to lay down without using as many pillows to elevate my chest and head. I began to see normal, slowly drawing closer and closer to my life.

The new norm was focused around traveling to Charleston twice a week. The doctor wanted to keep a close eye on my condition and respond quickly in the event of trouble. Thankfully, no trouble was had. I did require blood and platelets from time to time but no emergency sickness or infections. So week after week, we returned to Hollings Cancer Center, had blood drawn and infusions as needed, and then returned home for a couple of days before doing it all over again. And little by little, I could feel life returning.

Along with the reduction in my use of oxygen came a reduction of my dependence upon the wheelchair. I was able to use the walker within the home and even move some without it when I had something upon which to hold myself.

My heart seemed to stay in its normal rhythm and though weak was improving. The echocardiogram showed my blood flow through the heart to be only about 25 percent. Normal is around 70 percent. I had been assigned a cardiologist before leaving the hospital, and he was seeking to control the irregular rhythm and weakened condition of my heart through medications. A blood thinner, heart regulator, and water pill were used to relieve the stress upon my heart and keep it functioning though with less intensity. The result was frequent trips to the restroom, a good exercise program, and a frequent lightheadedness when getting up from bed or sitting. I had to adjust to moving more slowly and being careful to get up, get my balance, and be sure I was ready to walk before moving. On a number of occasions for the next several months, I found myself in transit from standing to crumpled on the floor when the lights went out. Thankfully, I was never hurt, but the reduced heart rate was a new normal that would last for many months yet.

It was a special Thanksgiving as my sisters and I gathered in my home to celebrate a continued life together. We, with our spouses, sat around a table laden with the traditional Thanksgiving food moved by the reality of how close death had come and how precious our connection as family was. We prayed, ate, laughed, and cried. We reaffirmed the bond of togetherness and departed with a hesitation to turn loose of a special time together.

Minor adjustments in treatment were being made, and the process was becoming a routine. The doctor had reduced my Bumex but found that I began retaining water again so we went back to the earlier dosage. I was showing positive signs of recovering from the chemo, and new hope was starting to build. My next trip to Charleston was only a few days away, and I would be there for another week for chemo once more. But once again, a dark cloud was descending upon our hope.

> Earl J and I traveled to Charleston this past Sunday for this month's chemotherapy. He had a 7:30AM Monday appointment for lab work, saw the nurse practitioner, and was to return at 2PM for the first chemotherapy treatment of the week. When we returned at 2PM for the infusion, we were sent to see the doctor. Remember that mutated FLT3 gene? Well, it reared its head. The doctor informed us that the leukemia blasts were back. So what now? Where do we go from here? The obvious and needed course is the transplant. Earl J's heart is still under the 50–55% ejection fraction (EF), but he is getting closer. The echocardiogram this past week showed his EF is up to 48%. The next option she presented was a clinical trial of a new agent ASP2215 (no name for the drug yet). A medication taken by mouth every day. It has been introduced to 23 patients. Earl J would be the 24th and MUSC's 4th patient. Results so far have been good. One patient's blast dropped 75% with the first cycle of treatment. The downside so far seems to be few, the major being eye damage, some fatigue, and lots of visits to Charleston since it is a clinical trial. Earl J asked the doctor about other options if he didn't do the clinical trial. "Go back into the hospital and repeat the initial chemotherapy treatments."

She did not want to do that due to the additional wear and tear on his body and heart. Unpleasant flashbacks for Earl J and I. We looked at each other and Earl J told her we trusted her knowledge and instincts. So he will be doing the clinical trial. The medication for the atrial fibrillation is not compatible with ASP2215, so it will be discontinued. Lab work showed it was messing with his thyroid anyway.

When I returned to receive my infusion, the nurse said, "Mr. Spivey, you need to see your doctor first." I could feel the darkness descending. That is never a good sign. So my wife and I walked down the hallway to meet with my doctor.

She explained to us that the blood test revealed that the previous chemo was ineffective against my leukemia. It was then that we were educated on the FLT3 genetic mutation. About 25 percent of acute myeloid leukemia patients have this mutation. It isn't for your benefit either. The nasty little mutation is quick to recognize what is destroying it and mutate to compensate for it. The doctors have witnessed it many times be nearly destroyed by a chemo treatment only to return with an immunity to that type of chemo. I had the worst of the bad, the FLT3 mutation. My doctor was very concerned about the matter.

As to the options available, only the very strong treatments I received in the hospital would be effective. To take the treatment again, I would have to be admitted into the hospital and undergo the seven days of one and the three days of injections of the other. But we all knew that would be a death sentence for me. I was getting stronger, but such stress would finish the weakening of my heart as well as the lung infection and other complications caused.

Our heads slumped and our spirits fell. We sat in honest conversation confronting the reality and not hiding behind any pretenses. The future was bleak to us, but there was one unknown possibility.

Some years earlier, someone decided to stage a chemical attack on the FLT3 mutation. Experiments were conducted, research studied, and a medication developed, which would focus on this mutation and stop it. It had just become available but only in an experimental use. It had been tested on animals but was just being approved for human testing. The uncertainties were all laid before us and no false promises made. It would be an experiment. Only twenty-three people in the United States had participated so far. The lab experiments with animals showed the two main negatives were deterioration of eyesight and heart function. Neither would be well tolerated in my condition.

Two choices were all I was given. One was sure death and the other unknown. I whispered a prayer, "Lord, you have carried me this far on this mission. I trust you to carry me into the unknown." And with that, we agreed to become the twenty-fourth patient in the experiment.

I was to stay another couple of days and do some testing to set a baseline of my condition, eyes and heart particularly, and then begin the experimental drug a few days later.

"Tuesday was a digest and reflect day, and maybe a couple of naps. Wednesday was baseline testing day. More lab work, three EKGs, an echocardiogram, chest X-ray, bone marrow biopsy, and a two-hour baseline eye exam."

My wife wrote:

> That was to become a routine for my visits. The drug would be taken on four-week cycles. The start of each cycle would begin with three EKGs taken five minutes apart. The eye exams and bone marrow biopsies would be stretched out a little more. About every six to eight weeks, a thorough eye exam was made and a bone marrow biopsy about the same time. I had agreed to participate, and my participation entitled me to free poking and prodding along with other benefits that brought more joy to my visits to Charleston. But that was the necessary pathway and self-pity or dread would not change it. Thankfully, pain was of little intensity.

The experimental drug would be taken as five pills first thing in the morning without food. They had to be taken one hour before eating or at least two hours after eating. I now added them to the thyroid pill that I had to take in the same way each morning. Every day began with six pills, an hour wait, and then something to eat to help protect the stomach from the handful of other pills to be taken. I had the three heart meds mentioned earlier, an antivirus, antifungal, antibacterial, and a few others as well. Anti-nausea meds were taken as needed and thankfully, they were needed fewer and fewer days.

I was now off the oxygen and rediscovering a good night's sleep. The wheelchair was parked and seldom needed. It was almost Christmas, and God had one special gift for us all.

> Our last visit, we were told that the leukemia blasts had dropped from 7% to 4% with the new drug ASP2215. Today, they said they found no blast. For this, we are thankful. His WBC, platelets, and neutrophils are still dropping, which is to be expected. He did not need any red blood cells or platelets today, another praise. The doctor stressed the importance of Earl J taking care not to catch anything.

"No blast." Was it true? Five months of battling leukemia and finally, it was no longer found in my blood tests. Needless to say, there was much thanksgiving and celebrating during the Christmas of 2014.

Some would say, "How lucky!" Others, "How fortunate that the new drug was available." But I think, more of how wonderful that the God I serve brought together at just the right time a drug and one in desperate need of help. This journey was not a sad walk through sickness. It is a journey in which God is showing His power and love to those who trust in Him.

Now would come the New Year. What would it hold? Still no insurance, still no progress in getting any. Still weak and in serious medical condition, but now with a new hope. It was to become a long and difficult year. But it would be a year of recovering and feeling human again.

With the starting of the experimental drug, the new routine was set. Each week, sometimes twice, I would make the trip to Charleston. Blood work would be run, and evaluation of my condition made. About once a month, an eye exam was done and a bone marrow biopsy about the same time.

The light of hope was beginning to shine. With the oxygen no longer needed, I had more freedom to move about. I still had to wear a mask and battle fatigue, but at least, I felt some renewed freedom. I could tell that without continuing to take chemo, my strength was beginning to return. The independent ways of living were being regained. By the end of January, I was getting strong enough to get out and move about by myself. It was at the end of January that a young lady my wife and I had known was killed while working at a convenience store. I was asked to help with the funeral and agreed to be present at the funeral, speak briefly but not go to the graveside. It was a very tiring experience, but it felt good to be able to participate in ministerial work again.

February saw a continued betterment of my condition. The biopsy and blood work showed that the leukemia was being held at bay. I was finally reaching the bottom of my blood system's damage from the chemo. By March, my blood numbers were starting to rise once more. Getting blood or platelets was very rare now. My system seemed to be moving back to a more normal plateau. I wondered just how normal that plateau would be.

By early March, all seemed to be going well. My red blood cells, platelets, and white blood cells were all returning to normal. That enabled me to go without a mask for the first time in five months. It was a joyful freedom to go out of the house and not have your face covered by a breathing filter. The returning to normal of my blood system gave me more strength. Another echocardiogram was done and revealed that the blood flow through my heart had risen to just under 50 percent. I still had to be careful with the lightheaded spells, but now they seemed less frequent and not as severe. With the warming of spring, it was time to get out of the house and stretch my wings again.

By April, I was able to write the following on the CaringBridge site.

> God is answering your prayers and blessing me with renewed strength. My good cells (red blood cells, white blood cells, and platelets) are all up near the normal mark. My leukemia cells are being held low. The experimental drug has been used of God to give me a breath of fresh air as I await the transplant. I am now free of the mask and able to ride the lawnmower and tractor some. Lauretta shares her wise counsel with me about not doing too much, and I do try to remember my medical condition. But with spring and a renewed energy, it is hard to hold back until I feel the continued weakness and remember.

I was starting to come alive again. I could now do lightweight jobs around the house. I could help with the house renovations for the ministry to single mothers. It felt great to do something physical again. Though I could not turn myself loose, I could return to many of the simple joys of working. And one more freedom came.

For several weeks, I had nurtured a rash around my PICC line site. It wasn't anything alarming, just annoying. We used some creams, but it would just come back. Now it was worse. It itched and was a constant irritation. It was great for the many times blood was drawn or infusions were needed, but otherwise, it was pain. To take a shower, I had to wrap my upper arm where it was located with plastic and seal it with tape. You had to be careful not to let it get wet or sweaty in order to avoid infections. The three connections dangled on your arm as you moved. So at a regular visit, the doctor looked at the rash and asked, "How important is it to leave it in?" By now, not much! I wasn't getting any routine infusions, and the drawing of blood could be done in the lab the old-fashioned way.

"Let's take it out then," he said. And with the nurse holding my arm still, he gave a firm pull and out came about eighteen inches of plastic tubing. A little pressure on the entrance site along with a tight bandage and I was good to go home. The rash soon cleared, and I experienced no more problems.

As soon as the hole in my arm healed, I had more freedom. I could take a shower without wrapping my arm. No more having to protect it from water. Now I could sweat and not risk infection. Now the dangling tubes were gone, and I was back to the old me.

The weeks slowly became months as the next few months passed. No significant change in my condition. I appeared to have reached the plateau. It was one of limited strength but freedom nonetheless to accomplish lightweight jobs. I was able to speak in churches when asked and work with the ministry I had begun. I could use the tractor to clean up and keep the grass in the pasture cut. I was able, with the help of a close friend, to make a workshop out of an old tobacco barn behind my house. My stamina wasn't lengthy and my strength not very strong, but I could finally work once more.

As the days and weeks passed, I had many occasions to reflect upon my illness and inner response to it. Let me share part of a CaringBridge post in which I shared some of my reflections.

> God is He who provides for His children and the glory goes to Him. Being patient and trusting has reached a much greater level in my daily living. It continues to bloom beautiful flowers of comfort and peace as I walk through the many dangers while feeling the comfort of God's presence in my life brings. Pray for God to continue His work in my life. Pray for me to have wisdom and strength to reject Satan's deceptive efforts to rob me of God's gifts to me. God is blessing more than I could have imagined. And my soul rejoices in the greater fellowship and meaning this cross of leukemia has brought to me. As Fanny Crosby, the great hymn writer, once said about the error that left her blind from infancy, she would not go back and change it if she could because her

loss was what brought her closer to Christ and made her the instrument she became. Wow! I can honestly say with her that if the absence of leukemia would leave me without the special things God has been doing in my life, I too would not change it for a more healthy life. I close with this thought that came to me the other day during a Bible study group, "One man's stumbling block is another man's stepping stone!" May God continue to keep me from stumbling so I can step higher and higher on His stepping stones for me.

The plateau seemed to have been reached. I could get out and work though lightweight only, drive, speak, move freely about the community, and do whatever I felt up to doing. Over the next few months, my strength would slowly increase but not very much. I was once more enjoying the freedoms of human strength and willful intentions.

In June, I put the following in a CaringBridge post.

As for now, I am using the strength I do have to push forward with Bethesda, the single mother's ministry. It continues to move forward though slowly. But after all, God is the keeper of time, and we are to live by His clock. I am also trying to tie up loose ends that I want to do before reentering the hospital. And so each day brings many thanks and joys for what God is enabling me to do.

The single mother's ministry, Bethesda for Single Mothers, is a story in and of itself. I had resigned my thirty years of pastoring to bring this God-given dream into reality. Too young to retire, not wealthy enough to be self-sufficient, and not sure how I was to financially survive, it became a great plunge of faith and exciting spiritual adventure.

The ministry was to take two houses received as an inheritance from my father's estate, one to me and the other to my sister, and remodel them to be used to house a houseparent and two girls who had just given birth. The two houses would enable us to minister to a total of four girls once completed. The idea was simply to provide a safe place for the single mothers to rebuild their lives once choosing to remain a mother to their child. We would walk them through their education, career training, and homemaking. We would over a four-to-six-year period of time take them from a frightened young mother to a confident godly mother able to be self-sufficient and a solid community member.

I began the work of renovating the houses and prayed for others to be sent by God to help in the work. I also prayed for the necessary funds to finance the ministry. I found four men with diverse skills and training needed for the oversight of the ministry and formed a board of directors.

It wasn't long before word began to circulate and people began asking to take part in the work. So individuals and groups began helping on the renovation and site-cleaning work.

God was moving on people's hearts to give financially to the work. We chose not to go the fundraising route. I admired the spiritual stamina of George Muller in England and Hudson Taylor in his Inland Mission to China. Both stated boldly that when God sends His servants, He provides for His servants. They both committed themselves to pray for God to provide the needed resources and refused to solicit contributions or gifts from others. And both found God's supply plenty enough for amazingly large ministries, Muller for an orphanage and Taylor for church planting in China. I was about to discover the same.

I would survey the needs and then kneel in prayer in the front room of one of the houses serving as the office space for Bethesda. As I sought God's gifts and pledged to give Him the honor and recognition for them, the bank account began to grow. It is now two years after the initial starting of the renovations and God has provided finances, supplies, work teams, individuals working on a regular basis, and so much more. None of which was asked for or sought after. It has been amazing to experience God's blessings and will continue to be so I am sure.

Now that I was able to enjoy freedoms and limited strength again, the awareness of returning to MUSC was an ever-present cloud over my life. I was now able to do things and therefore able to start preparing for the inevitable. While the Medicaid SNAFU of funding a stem cell transplant drug on and on, I was somewhat glad it gave me time to accomplish a list of things that I would like to have done, not knowing if or how I might return home.

July to November were months of almost normal living. I ran the tractor, worked with the men on the houses, spoke some in local churches, and worked on projects I wanted done before reentering MUSC. It was a great time of getting a fresh breath of life. I was able to run the chainsaw and cut wood for our fireplace. I could even carry an armload and help split the firewood with a hydraulic splitter, of course. I did swing the ax a little, but it was always out of my wife's sight.

With the starting of school, the familiar routines of family life returned. Returning to the soccer field for the fall soccer season in the community recreation league gave us regular outings. Finishing the project of turning an old tobacco barn into a shop and library for my books soon became a reality. My wife wanted a room for her card making work and storage room, so the upstairs was turned into her room. With these completed, my "do before returning to the hospital" list was completed. I now could enjoy another Thanksgiving and give thanks for the year I had at home and with my family.

It was at a routine visit to Hollings Cancer Center that we discovered my heart had gone back into atrial fibrillation. It wasn't life-threatening so they made an appointment with my cardiologist for a checkup.

When I went for the checkup, I was still in atrial fibrillation. It appeared that now I was staying out of my regular rhythm. The doctor decided to put me on a monitor for thirty days to learn just what my heart was doing and then respond to it. My condition was such that I had not known before when I was in atrial fibrillation. There were no chest pains, shortness of breath, or other indications of heart trouble. That was the only encouraging news. It seems that those who are not able to detect when their heart goes out of its regular rhythm are more endangered by the condition.

The monitor sent real-time info to a monitoring office. I found out someone was watching when I received a phone call shortly after returning home with my monitor. "Mr. Spivey, this is…"—and she gave her name and the company reading the monitor—"Are you feeling okay?"

"Yes," I said. "Maybe a little lightheaded but okay."

"Are you sure you feel okay? No chest pain, tightness in your chest?" She went on to add a few other symptoms. Then concluded our phone conversation with, "If you are feeling okay, then be careful." I agreed I would and said good-bye.

That was the first of many conversations over the month of December. On several occasions, I was awakened at two or three in the morning by a telephone call. It would be the monitoring agency. "Mr. Spivey, are you feeling okay?" I would struggle to get coherent enough to answer and muffle out, "I was sleeping fine till you woke me."

The operator would ask the familiar questions, and I would give the familiar answers. Sometimes, they would tell me what happened and sometimes ask me to push a button on the monitor that would send a recording of what my heart was doing. I learned early one morning that they were calling because my heart was stopping for an extended period of time. I never knew it in my sleep because it eventually started back again. But as was expected, my doctor wasn't very happy with the report.

Sometimes in the day, as I worked around the house, I would get the familiar call. One day in particular, I got a couple of calls. I had been using the chainsaw to cut some firewood and one needed some cleaning and adjustment. I gathered my tools and went behind the barn to avoid the oversight of my wife. I disassembled part of the saw, cleaning and checking it for needed repairs. I reassembled it and prepared to test it out. Two or three pulls on the cord and it still didn't run. A smart person with heart trouble and wearing a monitor would have disconnected it and let them think you were taking a bath. However, I've never claimed to be smart so my "mule-like" spirit kicked in, and I gave it a few more quick pulls. It was still not firing. I was breathless, and my arm was weak so after a moment's breather and a few more pulls, finally it started. I turned it off because I was so weak I couldn't safely hold it, and I was afraid my lights were about to go out. As I leaned on the tailgate of the truck, my phone rang. I didn't want to answer it because I knew who it was. But if I didn't, they might call 911, and I would have to hide from the ambulance. "Hello," I said. "Mr. Spivey, what in the world are you doing?" *What happened to "Are you feeling okay?"* I wondered. I tried to make it sound as innocent as possible, so I said I was just trying to start a chainsaw. "Well, stop it," the motherly voice said sharply. "Your heart is about to blow up."

"Okay," I said and promised to be good the rest of the day. A few questions and warnings later, the conversation ended.

I continued to rest a few minutes thinking that went over all right. Then the phone rang again. "Hello, I said wondering just who this might be?"

"I am," and she gave her name and continued, "a nurse in the cardiac unit at MUSC." Oh great, I thought now the monitoring company is a tattletale. She went on to explain that they had received the recording of my heart's hyperactivity and wanted to be sure I was okay. I assured her I was fine, just winded and an arm like a wet noodle but fine. "Please take a rest and stay away from the chainsaw," she said and concluded the conversation.

Needless to say, I pulled much less frequently from then on and better paced myself in an effort to avoid a duplication of that experience. I was glad that they didn't call my wife. I was able to humorize the situation and make it not sound so serious to her. I'm not sure she bought it though.

Christmas was soon upon us and a special time was had. Time with my immediate family was extra special being sandwiched in between my nearly fatal fight with leukemia and my soon return for the transplant. We enjoyed my extended family visits and my wife's family as well. It seemed a unique spirit was with us as we knew this was one more gift to us from the God who had given the world His Son.

As Christmas passed, our focus turned to a new year. My doctors had told me a couple of months earlier that it was time to do whatever I had the power to do to get medical coverage. The doctors saw some slight changes in my blood tests and were growing nervous that the FLT3 mutation was about to resurrect itself from chemical suppression. Thankfully, that never happened but with the lengthy delay, the doctors grew more and more nervous.

Shortly after Christmas, I was to meet with my cardiologist and discuss the results. There wasn't, however, much to discuss. My heart was staying in atrial fibrillation. No immediate danger of fatality, just the out of rhythm beating that promoted weakness and invited a stroke. The other problem for me was that no one was going to do a stem cell transplant for someone in atrial fibrillation. This had to be resolved prior to the transplant. We agreed on the course of action necessary and prayed for grace. And grace was soon to come in abundance and so amazingly.

Money Miracles

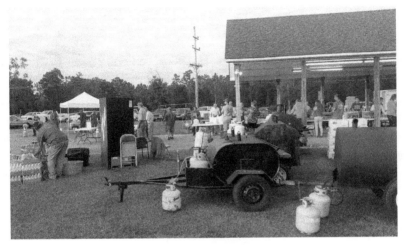

Benefit Preparations

After a day or two in the hospital, after the confirmation of leukemia in October at MUSC, dealing with the realities of life returned. My wife and I were blessed but not wealthy. We had an old truck and two cars, all paid for with no debts. We had one credit card with only a small amount of debt. Our only other bills were the mortgage, electricity, food, and other living expenses. I had taken some money from my retirement account to help sustain us over the last several months. But that was soon to run out. Now my wife wanted to be by my side, and the demands of caring for me and caring for our children made it almost impossible to work. So with a prayer of faith, we trusted the God who provides to show us the way.

Within a few days, people began to send financial gifts of various amounts to help us. Lauretta tried to keep a list and send out thank-you notes, but the list kept growing. We could not believe the generosity that was outpoured. Gifts came from people I had pastored, people from my home church as a child, friends who heard of my situation, and people I didn't know. Check after check flowed toward us because people cared.

There was the expense of gas for traveling, hotel rooms for staying when the children came with my wife, the continued living cost at home while my wife was no longer working, and other unexpected costs associated with my hospital stay.

We had always been an independent and self-sufficient couple. We took pride in managing our finances well and living within our own means. Now all this was gone with my diagnosis and hospital stay. We felt embarrassed and guilty for accepting other's gifts. We struggled to balance the great need we knew we were in and the inability to take care of ourselves, and yet, so humbled as people gave with such tender hearts and intense desires to help us.

We learned to thank God for the generous gifts of His children and yet refused to expect or feel entitled to such. We opened the cards laced with a check or cash and received from someone's hand their gift in love and were amazed at how God was providing for us.

It would be over a year and a half before I would be able to return for the stem cell transplant, previously known as a bone marrow transplant. In all that time, my wife stayed by my side and kept the home in place without working one single day. It was a miracle of God's kindness toward us. Here is how it took place.

The initial gifts enabled my wife to travel back and forth to the hospital and still meet the bills at home. She has always been very good at squeezing every penny out of a dollar, and now it paid off. Our little reserve in savings and what was left in our checking account was already getting low so we were anticipating another withdrawal from my retirement. That withdrawal never came.

Only after a few days in the hospital, I was visited by a social worker. She sat down and began to talk with me about my needs. Her first act was to sign me up for disability. I had never considered getting any assistance from Social Security under disability. She informed me that it would be well over a year before I could work so she would make application for me to get a disability check. That turned out to be $1,300 monthly. It wouldn't cover all our bills, but it would at least cover the mortgage and electric bill. Thank you, Lord!

As people gave, we put the money in my wife's bank account, and she squeezed each dollar to pay the remaining bills and any other unexpected expenses. There continued to be all that was needed, and never did we have to fret over unpaid bills or overdue accounts. The God who provides was meeting every need of His children.

Now for the really huge problem, the hospital bill! I knew that this wasn't going to be a free ride, and I was responsible for the hospital costs. Being uninsured was no excuse for not paying your debts. But I also know that whatever the final cost, you could sell all my belongings and me and my family into slavery and not come close to covering the cost of my stay and treatments. I could get well, and my wife and I could work for years and still only pay a small portion of the debt back. It was a dark cloud that hung in my room. A real test of faith to simply trust God to lead the way!

The social worker suggested that we try to enlist with Medicaid. If I was accepted, then Medicaid would cover my expenses and provide health insurance. So she gathered the information and began the process. She returned several times getting more information and clarifying some questions. Her supervisors finally concluded that I would not meet the criteria to receive Medicaid. The reason was that my wife and I had retirement accounts, and those accounts had way too much money to be accepted by Medicaid. Also, we had over $1,000 in our checking account and that was too much. So much for being careful about your expenses and saving for the future!

The social worker wasn't finished. She said she would try something else and maybe we could get help there. This continued for weeks and after six weeks in the hospital, we still had nightmares of a lifetime debt we would never be able to pay.

It was during the last week I was in the hospital that the social worker came into my room again. This time, she was smiling. "Mr. Spivey," she said, "we have another program within the hospital similar to Medicaid, and I made application for you in it. You are accepted, and it will cover all the expenses of your hospital stay."

I was speechless. Tears swelled in my eyes, and all I could say was, "Thank you, Lord!'

A few days later, I left the hospital not owing MUSC one cent. It was all covered, and the lingering nightmare vanished. My billing account sheet sent to me later revealed that my hospital bill was nearly $300,000 and sure to rise much higher. I still feel the emotion as I recall the grace of God upon this child of His.

It was shortly after returning home that one of the greatest money miracles occurred. I am recounting it as a third person because it was all done without my participation. It was the Earl J. Spivey Jr. fundraising benefit.

How it started, I do not know. I learned that members of the church I had pastored were meeting with a person familiar with fundraising efforts. The decision was to have a barbeque supper and have it on the church grounds. An outdoor shelter was there, and the church tent would be put up for those wanting to eat there. As I lay in the hospital, plans were being made for the event. It began to grow. My home church in Loris, sixteen miles away, sister churches whose pastors I had served alongside all wanted to join in. Individuals from the community asked to participate and before long, it was clear that this was going to be a huge undertaking.

The day was set. It would be a week or so after my arriving home from the first long stay at MUSC. That wasn't planned, but it just worked out that way. I wanted so badly to stop in and thank those cooking, serving, and helping for my sake. Medically and physically, it wasn't best for me to try it. I was still too weak, and I was warned by the doctors to limit my being around crowds of people. So I stayed at home and prayed for God's blessings upon those working so hard for me.

It was a beautiful day for a barbeque fundraiser. The cooks arrived the night before and began cooking the Boston butts in their large cookers. Those having prepared coleslaw, beans, and other sides brought them to the shelter. Workers arranged the plates, food, drinks, ice, and other elements for the meal as well as tables of crafts and items for sale. Within a few hours, plates were being served.

Some were delivered, and a spirit of unity and joy flooded the church grounds.

Churches of differing denominations were helping out. Individuals whom had never known each other worked side by side in jovial conversation. Crowds gathered at the tables under the tent, and the piles of barbeque and trimmings began shrinking as the people ate. There was plenty to go around and no one left hungry.

Tickets had been sold to help anticipate the number eating, but contributions came generously. Individuals would stop by for a plate and leave $100 for the cause. A couple even left $1,000 contributions. It was unbelievable. It was a special time when everyone knew God was moving among them, and it would be a time to remember.

A time to remember it was. I still hear comments about the unique spirit and joy that was upon all those helping. When the total was counted, just over $25,000 was made available to me as needed. I wept in disbelief of so many working so hard and so many giving so much for this small church pastor with no name. I was melted with appreciation and thanksgiving.

It was the benefit that would enable my wife to stay by my side and not work for the next year and a half. We stretched out the amount in monthly withdrawals to cover the bills not met by my disability check. And still others would send us gifts of money. Never did we go hungry or never even fall one month behind on any of our bills. The extra medical supplies and expenses were all met, and no financial stress was added upon my physical struggles.

To assure those who gave that the money was being used properly, a special bank account was created and Homewood Baptist Church, the church I had pastored, was given oversight. I would request the amount needed and a check would be given to me. No hassle or nitpicking was ever experienced, just a readiness to help my family through our struggles.

I was able to remain home for several weeks before having to return for another chemo treatment. As I would be treated in the Hollings Cancer Center, I would now have a social worker through them. She contacted us, and my wife and I went by her office to further investigate Medicaid. She asked for a few more documents and questioned us about how much money was in our bank account, retirement, and any other financial holdings. This took several months of conversation before she gave us her final conclusion.

I had left the hospital in October and now it was December. As she reviewed our case, she shared that her supervisors felt that I would not qualify for Medicaid. Though my bank account was now low enough, my retirement account was too much, and the benefit monies would be considered my assets so that would disqualify me as well. No application had been filed for me, and I had no letter of disqualification or denial.

We enjoyed Christmas together and rejoiced to see a new year. In January, I decided to call the government hotline and apply over the phone. The operator went through the questions and said I should hear something in about forty-five days. Forty-five days went by, fifty days, seventy days, one hundred days and still no letter. What followed was a long SNAFU, situation normal all fouled up, experience.

I would call the Medicaid office and another document would be needed. I would wait another month or two and no response. I would call again, and more information was needed. My wife stopped by to talk with a representative, and she said we were missing several documents. My wife told her we had sent them in and in a minute of picking at the computer, she found some of them. She assured us that only a couple of documents were needed and that a response would be given. So we dug out the documents needed and went to the Medicaid office in our county seat.

On the first trip, a document was missing so I was told to return with it. I was also told that a decision could be given when the document was received. So with anticipation of a positive decision, my wife and I took the document and went to the office.

It was now over a year from my leaving the hospital. Medical bills were multiplying, and the debt was overwhelming. I knew of no other options. If Medicaid said no, where else was I to go for insurance coverage? Shortly after being released from the hospital, I had met with my doctor. The plan was to get control of the leukemia and then move toward a stem cell transplant. The only problem for me was that the procedure was so expensive that the hospital wouldn't do a transplant unless some form of medical coverage was available. I had none so that is why the social worker was called in to help me. I didn't have a problem with the hospital's policy. Medical care was expensive, and I had no inalienable right to free medical care. I just grew frustrated with the lack of a decision and the mounting debt.

We were finally invited back to a representative and gave her the document. She took it, left the room for a few minutes, and returned. "Mr. Spivey," she said softly, "I'm sorry, but you do not qualify for Medicaid. You have too much money in your retirement account." I felt the teapot about to whistle. I restrained myself to only one comment. "But you knew from the start how much I had in my retirement account. You could have made a decision a long time ago." Now here we were over a year of hoping for help and waiting for a decision. The decision had come, and the answer was no. We slumped back in our chairs and struggled not to break out in tears.

After a few moments of silence, the representative asked, "You have a couple of children in school, don't you?" We said yes and told her what grades they were in. She said, "Let me check on something. Stay right here till I get back." And with that, she left the room again.

It seemed like forever before she returned. But she did and said, "I'm going to take you over to another consultant. She might be able to help you."

We were led across the hallway to another office and the representative greeted us warmly. We sat down and answered a few questions. She typed away at the computer keyboard and pushed her chair back and turned toward us. "Mr. Spivey," she said calmly, "because you have children in school, you qualify for another program that doesn't have the financial restrictions. You will get medical coverage under the program that is part of Medicaid."

"You mean I will get medical coverage through Medicaid?" I asked.

"Yes, sir," she said and then added, "since you made application in January of 2015, your coverage will start on January 2015."

I could feel the tears swelling up in my eyes. My hands were starting to tremble. The long ordeal was finally over. My medical expenses from January onward would be covered under Medicaid. No more waiting. The transplant was now possible.

I thought back some thirteen years earlier when God brought two children into our lives. We were both forty-five years old and feeling kind of old to start with babies. If we had adopted them just five years earlier at forty years of age, I would not be qualified for this program under Medicaid. I would still be without medical coverage. Coincidence or arranged by God? I believe that many of life's coincidences are divine arrangements, so I thanked God for His greater plan and arrangement.

It was a long trying journey that did more than challenge my trust in God. It once more showed me how God could reach into our past and remove what seemed unchangeable. Tears of thanksgiving and praise flowed time and again as the unbelievable became a reality.

I would still have the bill after leaving the hospital for October through December of 2014. That would be about $30,000, but what a small amount compared to the hospital stay and the year of medical bills while waiting for a decision.

As I write this, it is 110 days and counting after my transplant. My health is good, and God's miracles are evident. We have just used up all the benefit monies, and my wife has started looking for employment. I feel like the Israelites as they crossed the river Jordan. The Bible says that when they crossed the river Jordan, the manna stopped and the Israelites from then on lived on the fruit of the land. Now we are back to the fruit of the land.

People along the Way

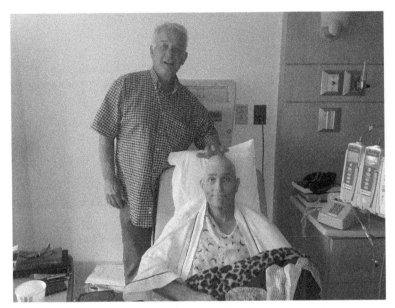

My Uncle from Florida

Somewhere in my development, I came to see life as a task-oriented journey. I was a dreamer and loved making my dreams a reality. I had enough self-confidence and ability to always find a way that if followed with a determined spirit would bring my dream into reality. The problem with that perspective is that people become objects to be used or moved about for the sake of the dream. I discovered after pastoring several years that my task orientation would have to be tempered with a more people-oriented perspective. I spent much prayer in seeking help focusing more on people and less on the achievement or noble accomplishments. One of those workshops was the Hispanic ministry.

Anyone who has worked among the Hispanic people can tell you time is unimportant to them. They are not driven by living on a rigid schedule. A familiar saying when the time to start a service or meeting has long passed is, "We'll start when everybody gets here." And once they start, they are not concerned with having an hour service and getting back to personal matters. "When we're through, we will leave." Bring a snack or even a meal because you never knew how long you were going to be there, unless us white folks were leading the service.

When I returned to South Carolina and pastored a rural church, I was asked by a nearby fellow pastor to help evaluate a spiritual response to the growing migrant population. The Hispanics were helping harvest the farm crops, and many were young boys working to support families in Mexico. They were given false promises and led to believe life would be easy and prosperous. That was the crew chief's story. He stood between the migrants and the farmers and, of course, got a significant cut of the migrant's paycheck. As the African American population was getting better educated, they were leaving the farm and taking less difficult jobs elsewhere. That left a vacuum for farm workers, and the farmers were turning to crew chiefs who would get the needed help for the summer season. The crew chiefs had their family with them, and a few of the workers came with their family too.

Our effort began with a two-pronged goal. One was an evangelical worship service where a couple of pastors would preach using an interpreter. We could not speak Spanish but began learning phrases and a few sentences.

Second was Club de Jesus or the Jesus Club in Spanish. It was a children focused time of music, Bible story, and just fun. We discovered that some of the children had to sit at the end of the rows in the fields where their parents worked every day. Others were left home unattended while their parents worked the fields. I visited the parents, and many came to the worship services and agreed for me to pick up their children for the weekly meeting of Club de Jesus.

Since I was musically gifted, I was designated to lead the singing during the worship times. I knew only two words of Spanish and no songs or choruses the Hispanics sang. I did my homework and discovered several choruses and short songs I could play on my guitar and that would be familiar to the migrants. One of my church members had a farm on which a migrant family lived. She loved children and agreed to work with the children while I and the other pastor worked with the adults. The husband of the couple living on her farm could speak limited English. He agreed to meet with me and help me learn to pronounce the lyrics to the choruses and sing their melody.

Over many years, I worked closely with the Hispanic people. I was honored to lead the church I pastored to sponsor the development of a Hispanic church, letting them use our old building we were using as a fellowship hall.

I would often meet with the Hispanic congregation to encourage them in worship. I would sometimes preach but had to have an interpreter, as I never mastered the language. It was there that God helped me to see the importance of the person and not the work.

As I waited for "everyone to get there" and stayed until "we were through," I was stretched painfully. I found God changing my driven nature into a loving nature. Churches come and go. Organizations rise and fall. Achievements are noted by plaques on the wall, but to care for others and focus on their benefit was a New Testament command I had overlooked.

What I had heard preached earlier began to take root in my thinking. "There are three things that last forever," at least according to the Bible, "God, God's Word, and the human soul." If I want to invest in something that lasts forever, it will have to be people. They are what really matter in life. As a result, my intense drive began to wane and my caring for people began to grow.

Now I found myself in the midst of a major illness. I believed I had been given a cross that would be used not to build some great work but instead to touch the lives of people. I would come to see that God would use me to touch others, but He would also use me so He could teach others to care about people.

It was only after a few days in the hospital that opening my eyes to focus on others came, and I knew to be alert and ready at all times. The evening nurse shift had come, and my nurse for the night came in to give me my medications for the evening. I remember so well this fairly young, attractive, and professional girl entering my room. I was lying in bed and turned to look at her and give her a word of greeting. I was struck by her stopping and just staring at me.

I had learned that sometimes when people have something going on inside, they will just stare for a few seconds to see if they really want to speak about it. So I just looked at her and let her stare. It seemed like a long time before she broke the silence.

"You're not afraid to die, are you?"

My first thought was, *And who said I was going to die?* But I didn't say it as I knew she was dealing with something important. I simply responded, "No, I'm not. I read the Bible, and I believe it tells me exactly what will happen when I do."

"Well, I am," she said.

For what seemed like ten to fifteen minutes, she released what had been tossing and turning in her heart for a year. She told me how her sister had died about a year earlier. She had several children, and my evening nurse had agreed to assume the mother's role. They were presently in another state with her boyfriend until she could finish her contract with MUSC and go to them. But every day, she feared dying young like her sister and worried about what would take place if that were to occur.

I shared a little of my faith's comfort with her and asked if she had a Bible. She had never owned a Bible and had not read from its pages. I asked if she would allow me to give her one. She enthusiastically agreed promising to read it. I told her I would get her one, and it would be hers to keep.

Over the next few weeks, I had the joy of giving her a copy of God's Word. I encouraged her to start reading in the Gospel of John and discover this Jesus Christ and what he revealed about Himself and our future. I rejoiced to see the heaviness departing from her face and voice over the next few weeks. She eagerly began to read and discover what only the Bible can teach us.

Another nurse named Jodie was a servant of God sent to comfort and encourage me. When she entered my room, I noticed that she was older than the vast majority of the nurses. I learned that she was there by choice to work among the cancer patients. I soon learned that she too was a follower of Christ. As we talked, I discovered that she attended the church that my friend from years earlier left Georgetown First Baptist to pastor. He was in a pastoral support group that I had joined.

She had a joyful spirit but firm medical direction. She had many years of experience working with cancer patients and still had a compassion to help each one whether they recovered or lost the battle. She had the brightest shoes. They were always a florescent color that almost glowed. Some were solid and some had patterns. I finally asked her one day why she wore such bright shoes when all the other nurses wore plain shoes. She answered that many of her patients would see her feet as she went about her nursing responsibilities. She wanted to brighten up their day and give them one more reason to smile and look on the bright side of their cancer experience.

God seemed to make a special connection between us that has lasted to this day. She always greeted my children and if they were not there asked how they were doing. If they participated in any special events, she wanted to see the pictures taken. She was a great comfort to me and help to my wife throughout this journey.

I would ask her about my pastor friend and how the church was doing. She would tell me how things were going. She also knew the pastor and told him I was in MUSC with leukemia. I was surprised when one day he came to visit with me and encouraged me in the struggle.

I noticed that she never seemed to work on Sunday. I asked her how she managed to always get Sunday off. She shared with me that it wasn't seniority or position, it was an agreement. She agreed to work each Saturday so she could be off Sunday to attend church and work in the children's area. I was moved to hear a fellow follower making a sacrifice of her Saturdays so she could be in worship on Sunday. I applauded her devotion and sincere faith. It wasn't about doing the church thing. It was about being in harmony with God and making the Sabbath of the Christian Faith a day of worship and service to God.

Throughout the year, between my post diagnosis and pretreatment, she kept in contact with us. She wanted to get the newsletters from the single mother's ministry and assured me of her prayers for me and my family. During each hospital stay, if she was not given me as one of her patients, she would come by to say hello and see that I was doing well before leaving. She always came with a smile and encouraging word for us.

While at home waiting for the transplant, she sent me an email. She wanted my perspective on prayer. She had seen the movie *The War Room* and wanted her preacher friend to share his thoughts on the concept. I encouraged her in experiencing the power of praying to God. I also shared with her that my focus in praying had shifted from a warfare to a time of worship. There was certainly a place in prayer for interceding for others and petitioning God for our needs. But the real focus in praying was a time of worshipping God each day. A time to humble myself to Him and prepare my spirit to guide my mind and heart in following Christ's will for me that day.

I noticed that she was a regular on the CaringBridge site. Almost each time I or my wife would post an update, she would leave us an encouraging word under the comments section.

She and I were talking after my transplant. I had shared on a post in CaringBridge about a burden I had to help lower income transplant patients. I wanted to call on the church and community to provide safe places for the transplant patient to get through the most dangerous time, a four-to-six-week period immediately following the transplant. She shared with me, "If I ever won the lottery, which I won't since I don't play it, I would use the money to build a place for the post-transplant patients to stay until they can safely return home." I could only say, "I pray that one day you will get the opportunity to do just that." Not by any foolish chance on a lottery but instead by contributors who will come together to financially meet a need that is literally condemning people to die.

Without any immune system, as it is destroyed by chemotherapy, the patients are sent home or to a local hotel where the conditions are neither sanitary nor emotionally encouraging to their recovery from such a severe medical procedure.

It was with much joy that after being out of the hospital a couple of weeks following my transplant, I felt strong enough to attend worship. My wife and I had no confusion on which church in the Charleston area we would attend. It was Jodie's church. I wanted to hear my pastor friend and also wanted to worship with my comforting and encouraging sister in Christ.

My family and I made the ten-mile trip from the hotel to the church and got there between Sunday school and worship. We went in, and Jodie's son and wife immediately recognized us. I was the only person there bald-headed and wearing a surgical mask. They told us they were under orders to look for us and seat us where their family sat. In just a few minutes, Jodie came from the Sunday school area and with open arms and a big smile welcomed us. We sat in the pew behind her and rejoiced to be worshipping with a special friend.

A couple of weeks later, we returned as we did for several weeks before returning home. This Sunday, they were going to observe the Lord's Supper. In the Baptist tradition, the plate of small pieces of unleavened bread are passed down each pew and later the tray of small individual cups of juice. This Sunday, I was sitting beside her with my wife on my other side. I was still having very noticeable tremors in my hands. I was concerned about handling the plate and tray with such shaking. As the plate was passed to me, I saw her hand reach for the plate and hold it for me to get my piece of bread. When the tray came later, she did the same thing again. Such was the heart of this nurse. She had a heart of compassion for others and cared greatly about the struggle others faced. She was a light for the dark days, a breath of fresh air on stagnate days, and a caring friend when all was going well.

Ruth came in pulling the blood pressure machine. She was dressed in black, MUSC's color for all working in her position. She was a tech or nursing assistant. They were responsible to check each patient's blood pressure, heart rate, temperature, and oxygen level every four hours. As mentioned earlier, they also check your weight every morning at 4:00 a.m. That was the glamorous part. They were also responsible to empty the bedpans when needed, measure the urine output and a few other bodily extractions. They made your bed and saw that you had as many blankets and pillows as needed.

She, like many others, was not from the Charleston area. Many of the techs and nurses came to work at the hospital from many other cities and states, even from other countries. Few if any of the techs worked in their position because they enjoyed it. Most of them, I was to find out were working their way up the medical staff ladder. Unable to go directly to college and earn a nursing degree, they first went to a technical college and received a quick degree that would allow them to start work as a tech and earn money. They would then take nursing classes during off hours to get their nursing degree.

Ruth's nature was joyful and pleasant. She was talkative and personal in conversation. As I talked with her, I discovered she was from the Midwest not far from where I had pastored many years earlier. She was dating one of the pilots from the nearby Air Force base. They were not too serious yet but were enjoying the bubbly joy of young love. Soon, her nursing studies would be completed, and she would graduate as a nurse.

We shared a number of stories from our lives and laughed much together. One came about during our discussion of meals. Somehow, I shared with her my dislike for liver and garden peas. She responded with her deep dislike for greens. Any vegetable that was green was refused by her lips, seriously!

When she was a child, her parents, like most parents, wanted her to eat vegetables. She didn't eat any that were green and leafy in particular. One night, the showdown came. Her mother fixed what her father thought was a delicious pot of mustard greens. As her father saw she was not going to eat them even after having them placed on her plate, he drew the line, "Young lady, you can just stay at the table until you eat your greens." With that, the battle was on.

Thirty minutes later, she sat quietly at the table. An hour later, she sat defiant and unrelenting. Two hours passed and the greens still sat on her plate, though now drying and appearing even less tasteful. By the third hour, it was getting late, but the staunch and determined heart held true. Sometime shortly thereafter, she fell asleep with her head on the table, and her mother took her to bed.

We laughed about the story and shared many one-liners about greens together as I saw her often when working. She was one of those "brighten your day" types of people. Even though I physically struggled through the eight-week stay following my diagnosis, I found a moment of refreshing lightheartedness when she was my tech for the day.

Like several others, I soon discovered she didn't have a Bible or have the custom of attending church on Sunday. We talked about the spiritual dimension of life and the importance of not being deceived into just living in the physical realm. I was able to give her a Bible that she would begin to read and discover Jesus's teachings about our spiritual nature.

Another of my nurses was from a faraway country. When she first came into my room, her height grabbed my attention. When she spoke, I immediately knew, "You ain't from around here!" She wasn't born in America nor did she speak English as her native language. As it turned out, she came from Russia.

I had to listen carefully to understand some of what she said. Her English was very good, but her heavy Russian accent caused her pronunciation of certain words to be much different than that of my southern dialect. She stood head and shoulders over the American nurses; however, she was just as compassionate and a very qualified nurse.

As you might anticipate, I asked many questions about her life in Russia. She was very warm and conversational as we talked of her life before and after moving to America. She had a husband, a fellow Russian, and two children. She always worked the evening shift so she could have as much time as possible with her children.

She did not meet her husband in Russia. Although he was Russian, they met in America, in Charleston actually. She had come to America through a recruiting effort by MUSC. She agreed to serve as a nurse for their help in coming to the United States. Her now husband had come to America to play basketball. One of the local colleges recruited him to play on their college team. As he was seven feet tall, they were glad to assist him in the arrangements needed to come to America. He played out his four years of eligibility but unfortunately didn't have enough hours to graduate. He wanted to stay in America and decided to return to school and get the degree needed to become a police officer. With a lot of hard work, he was able to get his degree and survive the police academy training.

Their paths soon crossed, and they began a relationship that would lead to their marriage. She was a nurse and he a policeman. They found a home and soon brought to it more life with two children. Life was stable and all was going well for these Russians living in America.

Yes, we soon began to talk of her religious heritage and experiences. She shared with me that she grew up in the Russian Orthodox Church. Her family was not very active in church life, but that was their religious identity. However, very close to home was an evangelical church she had attended from time to time and even made a commitment of trust in Christ as a child. For the most part, she had attended the Orthodox Church when she went to church in Russia.

Now that she had migrated to America, she had not participated in church. The Catholic Church was the closest thing to the Russian Orthodox Church in America. With no vibrant spiritual commitment, her church participation had been lost in the moving and establishing a new life in America.

One night, we were talking about our spiritual lives, and I asked her about returning to church. "You know," she said, "I was just talking to my husband before I came to work tonight about how we needed to go to church as a family." I encouraged her to take the big step of going to church for her and her husband's needs as well as the needs of their two children. I told her I would go with them if I could. I asked if she had a Bible, and she said that neither she nor her husband had a Bible. She wanted a Bible approved by the Catholic Church so I told her I would see that she received one.

I was very happy about two years later to have her walk into my room again during my transplant. We talked and revived our past friendship. As I talked, I was much disappointed to learn that she was still not involved in church. I had put her in connection with another nurse that was a devoted and faithful Christian. She had been invited several times and encouraged to meet this nurse at the worship service, but somehow getting there just never happened. I also learned that the person who was going to get a Catholic-approved Bible for her had never done so. I once again tried to encourage her to not let her spiritual life be left abandoned.

She was my nurse for only a couple of nights during the transplant stay. I didn't get to see her in the following hospital stays after my transplant. I still feel the sadness of how easy it is to just keep putting our spiritual lives in the closet. Our many good intentions somehow never turn into actions. Our inner awareness of what we need to be and do are treated as insignificant voices in the background of our minds, and life continues void of the spiritual meaning we were created to have. Others encourage and invite our participation in experiencing a spiritual fulfillment in our living from day to day. Until then, those of us living in the fulfillment that submission to Christ brings can still pray for a divine work that will help our loved ones push past the resistance that holds them back.

He usually came into my room in the shadow of the chief cancer doctor. When the chief doctor came around, he would lead a train of four to six others studying his profession. I say chief doctor because you didn't always see your assigned doctor. The hospital had a team of several doctors within the hematology diseases and cancer department. Every two weeks, the doctors on the floor and the doctors serving in the clinic would switch. Before I left, I had been introduced to them all. My assigned doctor would stop by at times even if she wasn't on the floor rotation.

This doctor was one of those studying to become a chief cancer doctor. Though he already had a doctorate in cardiology, he would still need several years of additional training and studying to become an oncologist. He wore the traditional white thigh-length coat identifying him as a medical staff with authority. He had earned the right to be an authority on matters of the heart but not yet matters of blood-related cancers.

Sometimes, he would make the preliminary rounds prior to the chief doctor's visit. It was then that we were able to talk on more personal matters, one, of course, being spiritual things. I soon learned that he was Catholic by faith. More so, he was a practicing Catholic. He often attended mass prior to his hospital shift and prayed for his patients. We talked often of our common faith experiences and the reality of our dependence upon Christ to guide us here as well as give us an eternal home.

I looked forward to those times when he could stop by to talk informally, and I think he made a special effort to come by so we could encourage one another. His long shifts gave us time to enjoy each other's company. He may be there for twelve hours during the day or all through the night. He was left when the chief doctor was gone to respond to situations that arose. So I got to see him often when walking the hall for exercise.

Though his strong faith was rare, it was an encouragement to me that there were others in the medical profession who not only drew on the spiritual but also actively participated in worshiping the God who relates to us all in spiritual ways. I was to discover that many of the nurses had a solid spiritual foundation. Some of the doctors accepted the reality of God's existence, and some chose to disregard it. But many saw through my life and others as well that when their efforts fell short, a mysterious something changed the medical prognosis that couldn't be physically explained.

As you can imagine, there were many unsung heroes who made my journey much more tolerable and refreshing. These were people who saw my needs and jumped to help without being asked. Here are just some of their heroic efforts.

I was the third in a family of five children. Oh yeah, did I happen to mention four of those were girls? Two were older and two were younger than I. We lived in a three-bedroom house on a small farm in northeastern South Carolina. Life was difficult on the farm. The house gradually became smaller and smaller. With five little ones between the ages of birth to nine years old, it was crowded to say the least. I can remember as a small child being crowded into one bed with three of my sisters so we could stay warm. I quickly became the "odd man out." I chose to sleep on a couch rather than be with the girls. When my two older sisters finished school and married, my two younger sisters took their bedroom and that left me with a room all to myself. The walls were painted hot pink, but that was fine as I finally had a room to myself.

We were a close family but had many territorial battles, and our natures were not always very compatible. Yet, we were family and as the old saying goes, "Blood runs thicker than water." There are many joyful memories of our years of growing up together. Though I saw myself as distinctly different and somewhat distanced from the feminine herd, I knew they cared much for me as their brother and were very proud of me.

As mentioned earlier, it was my oldest sister that accompanied us to Charleston when my wife told my sisters of my being sent to MUSC for leukemia. She encouraged us to allow my other sisters to help with the children and asked to go with us to the hospital. I was feeling too wasted to care, and my wife was straining to keep her nurse composure as we quickly accepted my sister's offer to be with us. We drove the twenty-minute ride to my sister's house and headed into the two-and-a-half-hour ride to Charleston.

By our side in the emergency room and up to the cancer floor she stayed, refusing to leave. She stayed the night with us and saw that whatever we needed was provided. She continued to make the long trips to Charleston to encourage me time and again, and she greeted me when I returned home eight weeks later. As you will learn further in this account, she was the one who was chosen to give to me my second earthly life. And now, my genetic fingerprint is hers and no longer mine.

Each of my sisters gave of themselves in unimaginable ways. For a week at the time, they would stay with my children while my wife and I remained in Charleston. They gave freely and generously to see that my children would not go without due to my sickness. My next oldest sister was faithful to give my children transportation to and from school as needed. One by one, they did whatever was needed for the moment to care for their brother. They visited regularly and transported the children whenever needed.

When I entered the hospital for the transplant, we all knew it would be three months before I would be able to return home. It was very humbling when, one by one, they took a week off from work and their routine lives to sit by my side in the hospital room or wherever I was to stay. They would read to me, laugh with me, and shed tears over the dark hours that seemed too heavy for me to carry. They had responsibilities to work and be with their husbands. Yet, whatever the sacrifice needed, they gave gladly to walk with their brother through the journey.

My sisters would often tell me, "If you need anything, just let me know." We often say that but don't really mean anything serious. While I was recovering from the transplant, my wife called me in the hotel to tell me that the washer had quit and wouldn't work. I had been an appliance repairman, so I asked for the details. It was more than likely the motor, and I wasn't able to repair it, of course, nor able to finance the repairing of it. We may have been able to purchase a washboard, but we would still need the tub. After much discussion and surveying the reality, I said, "Call my sister. Maybe she will be willing to help us with the repair."

My wife made the call, and my sister enthusiastically responded, "I'll come get you this afternoon, and we'll go looking for a new one."

My wife reemphasized that we only wanted to go the cheaper route, not wanting her to spend any more than was necessary. However, she insisted that she thought it would be better to replace it than to fix it, and she would be glad to take care of it. That after-noon, they went looking and when the looking was done, a delivery of a new washer and dryer was set for the following day.

My brothers-in-law stood in support of their assistance fully. Two gave their wives the freedom to be with me as much as they needed. The husband of one of my sisters, who was not physically able to make the long drive by herself, drove her to Charleston to spend the week by my side in the hospital. The other two brothers-in-law took a week off from work to sit by my side and drive me back and forth to Hollings. One came for a weekend and said, "You need a change of scenery. Let's go enjoy the weekend in a nice hotel." He knew that I just needed to get away from what was comfortable but had become a confining place. So I agreed and off we went, of course, still in Charleston. It was an all-expense paid weekend and no worries for me. We ate all the good stuff, and it was greatly refreshing to get away from the feeling of being trapped.

The negative side came Monday. He went back to work, and my sister replacing him took me back to Hollings as scheduled. The doctor checking on me asked me, "And how is your breathing?"

"Well…it is a little difficult," I replied. I went on to share our weekend exploits.

"You must have had a good time," he said, "because you have gained about ten pounds of fluid around your heart."

I knew what that meant. So off we went to the hospital for a couple of days of fluid removal. We joked about it from then on that I couldn't stand another weekend with this particular brother-in-law. But he showed the family support that was so important to my recovery.

Some years earlier, my uncle had retired and moved from Alabama to Florida. We had spent several vacation days with him and his wife renewing a brotherly relationship after years of going different ways. Being the youngest of my father's brothers meant he was still living next door to me for my elementary years. He would attend my football practices and encourage me in developing my sports ability, which was minimal at best. When he returned home from Vietnam, he would take me to the beach and treat me like a little brother. We enjoyed hunting together, so many afternoons were spent bird hunting on our small farm. When he started college, he returned to his enjoyment of sports. He played on the college baseball team. He would invite me to go with him and his girlfriend to the ballgames. During the summer, we decided to take a bricklaying class offered at the local technical college. Week after week, we would work the tobacco fields all day and then mix our mud, lay our brick wall and corners by night. We eventually received our certificate as apprentice bricklayers. The certificate is still kept and considered a treasured mark of our time together.

When he received word of my illness, he quickly called to offer whatever help he could give. To help my wife be able to return home and be with our children, he drove up from Florida to stay several days with me in the hospital. An even greater sacrifice was made following my transplant when he again returned but this time to stay with my children. It was a long week of taking the children to school, seeing that meals were provided, and he kept himself busy each day doing the many little things around the house that needed repairing and fixing up.

My cousin was one family member with whom a special bond was established. We had worked together growing up and spent a year together in college. After he returned home to finish his studies, our paths separated. We celebrated special times together and shared family grief. He had joined with me to help get the ministry to single mothers organized and running. When he learned of my hospitalization, he was quick to call me and knowing my outdoor lifestyle told me to not worry about the yard work. I had always taken care of the mowing. Week after week, he saw that the yard was cut and kept looking nice.

There were others who could not be by my side but expressed their love in other ways. One was my aunt. When she married my uncle, I was pastoring in a nearby town. She developed a close friendship with my mother. I would see her from time to time and somehow, she just felt close to me. On several occasions, when I would be strong enough to stop in and visit with my uncle, she would say, "Earl J, I want to give you something." She would give me a small envelope and tell me to use it wherever needed. It wasn't a small amount, however. Like so many in my extended family, she wanted to help and having the means to do so gave generously and freely.

There were many friends who also became my support team. Members from the church I had pastored, fellow pastors with whom I had worked, and acquaintances met over the years. Some traveled the three-hour trip to sit by my side and provide an encouraging support and assurance of their concern for me. Many gave to help us meet the expenses of travel, food, and the little things needed while away from home. Many others faithfully read our reports on CaringBridge. They would take advantage of the website to send me a note of encouragement. Each time we would send out another report, we would anxiously pull up the site to read what so many were sending back to me.

When my wife and I moved near my parents to become their caregivers through their journey with dementia, we built a log house to live in. Being an outdoor person who loved to camp and work out-doors, I chose to have a fireplace for our enjoyment and to help with the heating cost. My father had a couple of chainsaws, the ones that got me in trouble with the cardiology nurses, so there wasn't much of any expense in getting the wood. I did insist on getting a small hydraulic splitter for wood chopping.

As my weakness carried into the winter, we could burn what was already stacked. However, the following winter would not be so abundant. I was not able to do much cutting and though I had a friend to come help split and stack firewood, more was needed. I resigned to turning up the thermostat and paying a bigger electric bill. On a number of occasions, I would look out to see members of the church I had pastored coming up the driveway with a truckload of firewood. It was cut, split, and ready for the burning. On other occasions, I would see someone I did not know pull up to the house with a load of firewood and ask if this was my house. After affirming that they were at the right place, he would tell me that someone had bought a load of wood and told him to take it to my house so I could enjoy it. Time and again, I would come to tears over how those who knew me would support me during this difficult journey.

There were many people and churches that assured me of their continued prayer support. Cards, letters, and notes would come affirming that I was never forgotten but constantly in their prayers. One church was especially diligent. Pleasant Hill is a rural church near my home. They had a prayer ministry team that prayed for indi-viduals and groups regularly. With the consistency of the clock, I would receive an envelope with a prayer card enclosed. It was encour-agement to me from them that I was consistently being held up in prayer. I have always wondered who the team was but gave thanks for their faithful commitment to intercede on my behalf.

There are so many stories of kindness and compassion that car-ried me through the journey. All were God's gifts of kindness through human hands, hearts, and voices to support my weak tottering spirit. Thank you to all reading this book who have been one of the unsung heroes that made my unbearable journey bearable.

The Transplant Journey

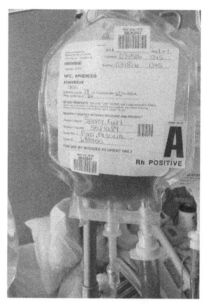

Millions of Stem Cells

It had been over a year since returning home. It was now early January, and my wife and I were to meet with the Medicaid representative. As shared earlier, we finally completed the documents wanted and were given medical coverage through one of the programs under Medicaid. The tears shed at the finality of being covered were twofold. First was the joy of getting help with the ever-growing medical expenses. Back dating the coverage to the application month of January 2015 was an unexpected gift. Tears of joy and thanksgiving trickled down our cheeks.

Second, though, were tears of heartache. Some weeks earlier, as the conclusion of our application for help appeared to be getting near, I began to feel the dark cloud and emotional weight of having to return into the "Gethsemane" of medical suffering. I now knew what was ahead. I had walked the pathway of chemo treatments. I had tasted and almost choked on the side effects of such powerful and life-threatening drugs. And yet, I had walked in God's peace and trusted in His care. Now it was time to return and with the gaining of medical coverage, the door swung wide open.

With mixed emotions and a flurry of thoughts, we returned home from the Medicaid office. We began trying to turn the mental corner in our minds toward the transplant. But first was the heart issue.

We met with my cardiologist about the next steps. He proposed that I enter the hospital the last week of January to have a cardioversion, an electric spanking of the heart, that would correct it from its abnormal rhythm. I was to remain in the hospital for a couple of days to be under observation while a regulating medication was being given and adjusted. I would enter on a Wednesday and return home by Sunday. That was the plan.

For the most part, the plan worked well. I entered the hospital, was prepped for the procedure. and was fast asleep before I knew what was happening. I awoke with my heart in its proper rhythm and beating strong. I was soon moved to the cardiac floor and made ready to start the regulating medication. By Thursday evening, things were not feeling so well. The chosen medication was causing me to be nauseated. I said chosen because the transplant team was now working with the cardiologist in preparing me for the transplant. An old drug that had been effective for me in the past was not available due to its interactions with the drugs used during the transplant. Back and forth they went in discussion until a heart regulating drug was found that would be acceptable. Here we were with two choices left, and one was having adverse and intolerable effects. Friday, the decision was made to stop the medication.

Starting the second choice was not as simple as just taking another pill. The first medication had to be out of my system before the second could be started. It would take at least twenty-four hours for the first medication to leave my system. I would have been allowed to return home for the waiting time and then return but not right now. The hospital was very busy and filled with patients. The doctor was concerned that if I was discharged when I returned the next day, a room might not be available for me. So, I was kept in the hospital to wait. Saturday came and went and Sunday arrived, the day to start the second and only option.

I started the medication and the EKGs soon followed. Routine EKGs were done to evaluate the effect of the medication on my heart. They revealed that the dosage was too high, and they adjusted it until I was at the lowest dosage. The three days went smoothly with no side effects noticed. With the proper dosage found and no adverse side effects seen, I was at last free to return home again. CaringBridge entry:

> I have returned home again, though briefly. The last two days have been more than amazing. As goes my heart meds, we finally settled on Tikosyn to help regulate the heart and help me stay out of atrial fibrillation. The doctor reduced it twice so I take it at its lowest dosage. The sickness is almost gone completely. So, last night, we made it back home. And now the last two days. They have been days filled with great emotions and staggering information. Days where the hand of God upon my life is evident and visible. My sisters were told that the possibility of them genetically matching me and being a donor was no more than about 25%. So we were encouraged to not be disappointed but look instead to the national donor bank. Monday afternoon, the bone marrow transplant team coordinator called to let me know that my sister just younger than me was my perfect match. She will shortly begin the process of becoming my donor. I could only weep and thank God for His kindness and amazing work as to let my sister be the giver of new life in me. With that crucial piece of the puzzle in place the wheels began churning quickly. Tuesday morn-

ing, Lauretta, Christine, and Elliott came to meet with the social worker on the BMT team and take me home. The social worker walked us through many questions and shared much about the transplant experience. We were to meet with the BMT coordinator at some later date. So we checked out the hospital about noon and headed over to Hollings Cancer Institute to meet with the doctor. Before the nurse practitioner came into the room, a young lady came in and introduced herself as my BMT coordinator. She sat down and for about an hour walked us through what was ahead. As we listened, she talked of the many things that would take place. And then said, "We have a target date for your entering the hospital on February 24th." I could feel the wave of emotions crashing upon me as it was no longer sometime in the future but now just 3 weeks from now. So the rush is on. So many things to do before returning. The transplant will require that I say in Charleston, or Mt. Pleasant most likely, for 3 months. If I am one of the fortunate 50% who survive the transplant, I can expect to return home about June. Most of the time, I will be in isolation to prevent any viruses or infections. And time and again, I will be rushed back to the hospital for medical help. Soooooo, here we go. Through many emotions and rushing to do many things before leaving home again, I now walk the journey. But God is my Shepherd, and I rest in Him.

As I remember that day of which my CaringBridge post just described, the emotions still flood over me. The transition was happening so quickly. The reality of what was about to take place was difficult to grasp. The emotions of joy in the future hope, fear of the real dangers, heartache of the coming suffering and sadness of leaving home again all swirled within me.

My heart was now ready for the journey but was my real heart ready for the journey? I was physically in the best shape since the diagnosis of leukemia. But, was I strong enough to withstand the chemo and physical stress? My faith was strong, and I was grateful for God's word to me and help over the past year. But, was I ready to leave my family and world behind for the greater joy of a heavenly promise? Now the reality slowly settled in. No more pushing it aside with some day in the future. A mark was on the calendar, and the countdown had begun.

Grace in abundance was about to flow. The day after returning and writing the above post, I received another call from the BMT coordinator. "Mr. Spivey, I am excited to tell you that your oldest sister also tested as a perfect match for your transplant. Since she has never given birth, the doctor wants to use her."

My younger sister had given birth to two boys. They explained that when a woman gives birth to a child, certain antibodies are created in her system. Those antibodies could create greater difficulty in the transplant by rejecting elements in my body. So the doctor chose my older sister to avoid the risk of rejection.

Of four sisters, two tested a perfect match, ten out of ten markers used. God had blessed in abundance. My younger sister was disappointed but was glad I would not be exposed to the antibodies childbirth created. My two other sisters were disappointed that they had not matched because all were eager to make whatever sacrifice was needed to give their brother life. That was the greatest blessing given. My oldest sister rejoiced to be the chosen one and was ready and waiting to begin the process. Two perfect matches and two others that were very close has to be a record!

After another meeting with the BMT coordinator who shared the reality of a stem cell transplant with me, I wrote the following.

> Saw the coordinator and she gave us the gory
> details of the transplant. It would make the weak
> of heart faint and the courageous run. Were it

not for the fear of dying, few would dare the journey. But I believe the God I serve leads me along this pathway and will be my comfort and strength. So onward into the jaws of death and great suffering not for the hope of life but in submission to Christ and in hope of being His chosen instrument.

It may not have been quite so frightful, but it was scary. The coordinator was honest and wanted me to know exactly what was ahead. My decision had to be final and lasting because once the chemo was given, there was no turning back. I would then have to be ready to face whatever came out of the mysterious and dark unknown. No promises, no pledges of desired outcomes, and not even any assurances that all will turn out all right.

There were many risks and multiple dangers. From lasting medical conditions that slowly take your life to sudden breakdowns that take your life quickly, I had to be ready to face them. There is good reason that only about half of the transplant patients live to see the hundredth day following their transplant. And of those, only about 50 percent will celebrate five years later. It is a brutal form of healing. But the only other option is to be medically comforted and die. It is a fresh picture that in hope of living, we will endure great risks and suffering. How precious is life to us.

As a Christian, life is more than this earthly existence to me. I believe that Christ gives me an eternal state of existence because I accepted His invitation to be part of His family. Yet, I had pastored for many years and witnessed many of the faithful shudder in fear at the prospect of dying. But I have seen many others walk into the darkened fog of death with confidence and joyful anticipation. I wanted to be one of the latter. I was headed into "the valley of the shadow of death" and needed to be ready. I had no assurance that I would arrive home alive or continue the meaningful experiences of life here on earth. I reached deep for confidence in my faith and sought God's comfort to walk wherever this pathway led.

There were still, however, a few physical hurdles to jump over. My heart needed a little longer time to prove itself. I was given an appointment with the cardiologist for the week before the target date. Meanwhile, I had to visit an oral surgeon and have my teeth checked and any with infection to be removed. A scary thought for me. I had not been to a dentist in nearly forty years. My last visit had been a nightmare for me, and I had no intention of returning until the cure hurt less than the illness. An appointment was made at the MUSC dental school and fearfully I went.

My wife and I arrived at the waiting room somewhat early following a visit at Hollings. As we waited, the rather large waiting area began to fill. I was soon called back and made more nervous by the arrangements. As a teaching institution, the dental school did a large volume of work. The many dental students were moving about practicing their instructions. As I walked behind the door, it led into a long hallway. On the left was a series of cubicles separated by curtains. There must have been twenty of them, one after another down the left side of the hall. *Pain chambers of torture and suffering*, I thought as I passed by them.

On the right side of the hallway were rooms for diagnostic and gathering purposes. One of them was the X-ray room. I was taken in it and told they would do a complete X-ray of my teeth and gums. I was given a lead apron-like garment to wear over my clothing. It covered my chest, waist, and upper legs. I was led to a contraption where I could bite on a plastic looking piece in front of me while standing. On both sides of it were two flat things I assumed made the X-rays. I bit on it and was told to remain still while the two flat pieces moved around my head. Around my head they went, and the X-ray was done.

I was then taken to one of the cubicles and invited to make myself comfortable in the chair. How ironic to get comfortable before being tortured? I settled in the chair in fear of what the X-ray would reveal and the dentist, or student, would do. The student came in and was pleasant. He poked and prodded in my mouth and asked a few questions. He said that doctor somebody, a name that let me know he wasn't from my hometown and probably not very sympathetic to my kind, would soon be in to see me. I sat nervous, wishing I had brought my Ativan with me.

Shortly, the doctor came in, introduced himself, and sat on the stool beside me. He was surprisingly gentle and pleasant in conversation. He looked in my mouth sat back and said, "Well, Mr. Spivey, the X-ray shows no cavities or decay. Your teeth are in very good shape, and you are clear for the transplant." I about wet the chair with excitement. No drilling, filling, pulling, or cutting. I was good to leave and make ready for the transplant. All I could think of was, *Thank you, Daddy!*

My mother had the bad teeth. Visiting the dentist was a regular for her. Daddy on the other hand never went to the dentist. He died at eighty-nine with all his original teeth still in place and no fillings that I knew about. With great rejoicing, I left and headed back home relieved at yet another gift of grace that enabled me to avoid further trauma at the hands of a dentist.

The next hurdle would be scary. It was the psychiatrist. Before taking someone through a stem cell transplant, the doctors want to be sure their patient is stable enough to withstand the mental stress of the process. The transplant team includes a psychiatrist to evaluate the patient's mental condition. I anticipated a lengthy test to be filled out and an extended conversation. And that it was.

The tests would take over an hour to complete. I sat in the waiting area so familiar to me at Hollings answering the questions as we waited to meet with the psychiatrist. Just before I had completed the tests, the psychiatrist came and invited my wife and me to a meeting room. No couch, just a table with several chairs used for meetings and dining. She had a psychiatry student with her that would be observing our interview. To my surprise, she was pleasant to talk to and didn't fit the weird mold often associated with psychiatrists. She didn't delve deep into my thinking, mental concepts or childhood upbringing. She was most interested in the family support and my realistic expectations of what was about to take place. We talked for forty-five minutes or so about my having gone through the difficult diagnosis and road to remission. We talked about my faith and its impact upon my handling of the previous stresses. We examined my family's rallying around me throughout this experience. When she seemed satisfied, she took her assistant outside for a consultation and returned. She gave me the green light to go ahead with the transplant, assuming no major surprises were revealed in the tests. And there was none, and the last major hurdle was now safely cleared.

The transplant team needed a little more time to evaluate the interactions of my heart medication, Tikosyn. The pharmacist on the team was not sure that it would be compatible with the other medications used. The new target date was set for two weeks, and I was not disappointed. Two more weeks to be home with the family and finish the little things I wanted to do before entering round two.

From this point on, everything carried with it the eerie feeling that this might be the last time. I hoped and prayed for more years to enjoy my family and continue the ministry I had started. I asked for more time to fulfill some things I believed God had started through me. Yet, I had no claim to a unique or special protection from God. I could just as easily be numbered with the 50 percent that didn't survive the transplant as the ones that did.

I talked honestly and frankly with my wife. We agreed how my possessions would be distributed if I didn't return. We shed tears and affirmed our trust in He who holds life and death in His hands. In life or death, we were committed to follow our Lord, and now was the time to prove it.

One of the most moving times for me was a tractor ride. I lived on the farm where I grew up. Until I graduated from college, I worked in the fields that now surround my log house and hunted the woods around them. I left after graduating from college, anxious to make my place in the world. The old family farm had little tug on my heart. But with time, that changed.

When I moved back to South Carolina from Indiana, I pastored a church close enough that I could visit my parents and help where needed during my parent's retirement. And when I was in between churches for a nine-month period, I stayed in my grandmother's home while helping my uncle on his golf course. Then I moved thirteen miles away to the last church I pastored, still regularly returning to parents and an old home place.

When it was time for me to move back to the home place to help care for my parents, I began to notice the change. As I would take over the running of the tractor to keep the farm trimmed and cut, I could feel a change. My father was no longer able to drive the tractor or keep the pasture cut and the ditch banks cleaned. He handed down to me the responsibility of caring for the old home place. But he had handed down to me something more.

My grandmother's father bought the farm in the early 1900s. I do not know the story of his acquiring it but when my grandfather was stationed in Virginia to catch moonshiners, my grandmother was given the farm and moved over from a nearby town. My father had grown up on the farm. When my father was still in high school, my grandfather returned from Virginia and started a dairy, and my father worked delivering milk and butter to the town close by. I was to learn just before my father's death that he had not planned to farm for life. He planned to get a job in a local town. It was then that my grandfather, who had retired by then, and my grandmother came to see him and asked him to return to the farm. They offered to give him the farm if he would assure them that he would build a house for them and give them part of the money from the crops. He was the son chosen to take care of his parents during the closing years of life, and he fulfilled his obligation willingly.

In 1954, my mother and father moved back to the farm and built the house in which my sisters and I grew up. I began to feel that I had become a part of a rich heritage. My grandmother cared for her parents on this farm until they died. My father cared for his parents on this farm until they died. I had cared for my parents on this farm until they died. Now, by God's grace, I wanted to be on this farm till I died. Of all the places on this earth, even with their beauty and amazement, nothing captured my heart like this ninety-acre plot of land. I had been handed down a place to call home. Not a place where I lived, but a place that was part of me, or perhaps me a part of it.

It was with all this moving within me that I prepared to do one thing left before entering MUSC again. I put on my old straw cowboy hat and work clothes. I went out to the shed and climbed up on the old tractor. With the sweet churning of the engine, I started around the farm. I went slowly around the perimeter of the home place. For me, it was the "homeland." As the tractor slowly made its way around the edge of the field, my eyes grew wet and my mind replayed many scenes from the life I loved here. It was my farewell tour around the farm. If I didn't come back to my beloved homeland, I had said good-bye and thanked God for the privilege of living on this small but most favored place on all the earth. I returned to the shed, turned off the tractor for what might be my last time, looked around slowly while wiping my eyes, and now I knew it was time to leave.

While I was preparing for my return, my sister had some preparing to do as well. She had to get a physical, answer a lot of questions, and make several trips to Hollings to meet with doctors and other medical staff. She had to give lots of blood for testing and prepare her mind for the discomforts ahead.

The stem cell transplant is much easier for the donor than the old bone marrow transplant. Before the bone marrow would have to be extracted from the bones, now that would no longer be needed. No surgery just shots, though painful they were, followed by a process called apheresis. The donor was given two Neupogen shots for about five days prior to harvesting stem cells. The shots would put the bone marrow in hyper drive and result in a glut of excessive stem cells. These newly birthed stem cells would be forced out of the bone and into the blood system. Once the blood system was flooded with these new stem cells, they could be filtered from the blood and infused into the recipient. To remove them, a needle was placed in one arm to draw out the blood. The blood would go through a separation machine that would separate the stem cells from the other blood components. It was a system based on the weight of the various components, the stem cells being the weightier. Once separated, the stem cells would be collected, and the rest of the blood returned to the donor through a needle in the other arm. Great theory, tough execution!

The process would take five to six hours. Once started, there was no stopping till the harvesting was complete. That meant very difficult potty breaks. Your two arms were immobilized for the duration of the procedure. If your nose itched, you better have a close friend nearby. If your nose was runny, then the nursing staff would delegate the undesirable necessity to the lowest ranking person. You can't even get a friend to do that. Well, maybe. My sister had her husband by her side all the way. He rubbed, scratched, and consoled his wife through the five-hour procedure until she could scratch for herself.

The worst of the ordeal was afterward. With the excessive demands upon the body and the stress of forcing the stem cells through the bone tissue in an accelerated manner, pain was sure to come. The next couple of weeks following the harvesting of the stem cells would leave her drained, sore, fatigued, and all around exhausted. So, it was nowhere near back to normal the next day. It would take weeks before feeling normal again. The stress induced would leave many achy joints and sleepless nights until the body could recover.

If about five million stem cells were harvested, once will do. If not, then the shots continued, and the procedure was duplicated the following day. My sister was one of the unfortunate ones. She had to return the second day to give more. The amount for both days was plenty with several million more frozen in case they would be useful later.

Besides the many trips to Charleston, the procedure would require my sister to spend the week in Charleston as well. The shots had to be taken at Hollings and given by their staff. Traveling back and forth every day was too demanding. She and her husband came to Mt. Pleasant, next to Charleston, and stayed for the week. She was to start the shots the day after I checked into MUSC. That way, the stem cells would peak the day of my transplant.

All the loose ends were being tied up and various matters finalized. The check-in date was now only a week away. One of the last posts before entering the hospital contained this account on CaringBridge.

> Yes, a long day. Had last eye exam about 11:00 today. Dilated my eyes and found no detect-

able change due to the experimental drug. Had a chest X-ray and it was clear, except for extra-large lungs. No comment there. Gave 13 tubes of blood in the lab and went to see the doctor. Saw the representative from the clinical trial, experimental drug, for the last time and had the last EKG. Met with the BMT coordinator to go over final details and sign necessary consent forms. Had one more bone marrow biopsy...

The last visit to Hollings was a planned infusion. Before I took chemo again, the doctor wanted me to have an infusion of a drug that would help give a big boost to my immune system. The immune system was going to be destroyed, of course, but until then, the doctor wanted all the strength I could get to ward off any infection or viruses near me. It took several hours and had certain side effects. As a result, many could not take the full dosage. The nurses kept a close eye on me and were prepared to stop the infusion at any sign of severe side effects. The side effects didn't take long. The familiar fatigue, achy muscles, chills, and all-around discomfort began showing up before we returned home. When I came in the door, I wanted a comfortable spot in the most out of the way place and to be left undisturbed. Thankfully, it was short lived.

March 9 arrived quicker than expected. The check-in date was here. The ride back to MUSC was quiet and full of reflections. Memories of the long road to recovery from my initial treatments replayed in my mind. Thanksgiving for the year just completed at home broke through the solemn moments of joy. Dread of what lay just ahead cloaked me like a dense early morning fog. But there was the comfort of my faith. I had been given a cross. That cross would be an instrument God would use in the lives of many others. How could I hesitate or refrain from the journey? My only choice was to be the best instrument for God He would want to use. It was with a commitment to press forward and give my best in the struggle that I entered my room and settled into my bed.

First came the flurry of check-in activities, blood pressure, temperature, heart rate, weight, and more. Then I was given a little time to regroup. I needed to prepare myself for the insertion of a subclavian IV line that afternoon. The PICC line was out and now, another access to my blood system had to be made. This time, a subclavian IV line was going to be used instead of the PICC line.

I was taken to the operating room about midafternoon. The doctor and a couple of assistants greeted me and assured me the procedure would not be painful. A localized numbing would be enough to avoid any pain. I would only feel a slight tugging and moving as the tube was threaded under my skin and into a main vein in the side of my neck. I remained calm as the doctor numbed the area and began the pushing, pulling, and pressing on my upper chest and lower neck. They stopped a couple of times for an X-ray to be sure all was where it was supposed to be. In just a few minutes, "All done," the doctor said, and I was quickly taken back to my room. That was the last preparation needed and the next morning, it would be chemo time.

> Yesterday, got things off to a bumpy start. The insertion of my chest port went well. I was quickly taken to my room. But soon, the nausea began to swell. I think it was mostly due to meds used during the procedure. I felt better later in the afternoon and better still this morning. So here we go my friends and prayer companions. Two closing coincidences that underline God's presence through this journey. First was my morning reading in Psalms. Several months ago, I asked God to give me a passage for this journey. He gave me Psalms 84. Guess which psalm was the one for today. Yes, Psalm 84. Thank you, Lord, for your reassuring. Several weeks back, a pastor gave me a daily devotional he had written. I set it aside to use once I entered the hospital. Today's devotional, my first, was focused on let-

ting Christ's light shine through our interactions with others. Again, God confirms I am on a mission. He has, is, and will be working through this frail servant. So here we go. Let's see what God has in store.

It was Tuesday morning and I had been awake since the four-o'clock weigh-in. I had spent time in prayer and Bible reading. I needed the inner momentum as we would start more chemo. This time, I would not be tied to an IV pole. The chemo would be taken in IV form but would last only about thirty minutes each day. The chosen chemo was Fludarabine. It would come with all the familiar side effects including the loss of hair again. "God, help me walk this valley just one more time please." I whispered as the IV was started. It was nine fifteen, and the transplant journey now officially began. My new calendar started with today as −5. The countdown was to the transplant day, day 0. That would be my new birthday they told me. On that day, your old blood system would be nearly destroyed, and the new stem cells once developed would finish the work of destroying what remained. The day after the transplant would be day 1, the first day of my new life. Since my sister's blood type was the same as mine, I would keep my blood type. Had hers been different, I would have her type hereafter. It was not uncommon for transplant recipients to come out of the process with a new blood type. After all, the stem cells will only produce the blood type they were genetically wired to produce.

Another interesting fact relates to the genetic makeup. Now that my blood system was destroyed and my new one was an extension of someone else's, I have their genetic fingerprint. If I committed a crime and the investigators found a drop of blood I had left and tested it genetically for an identity, guess whose identity comes up, yep, my sister. There's a lot of possibilities there. Hmmmm…

There is also some powerful imagery to be seen there. As I mentally prepared for living the rest of my life on the extension of my sister's blood system, the spiritual analogy was too strong to ignore. I believe that Christ's death on the cross paid the price of sin that I could not pay. I also believe that as the Bible teaches my life is no lon-ger mine, Christ's Spirit has come within me, and the life I now live is a new and different life from the past. I had practiced it and taught it for many years. Now I was experiencing a living symbol of this great spiritual truth. Though outwardly I was physically the same, inside I was physically changed. It was not my blood that gave to me life, it was my sister's. My life would now be evidence of the existence of someone else's blood within me, I am living. Without her blood, I would die. Without God's Spirit coming within me, I am spiritually dead. But thanks to the merciful God above, I have a new life to live under the authority of His Son. I would find the analogy regularly circling through my thoughts.

Day –5 and the process had begun. After the thirty minutes of chemo, I was free to move about the room and walk the hallway at will. Day –4 and no side effects as of yet, I ordered my meals and enjoyed the taste, not knowing just when they may vanish again.

Day –3:

> Today was the third day of chemo. I have been given Fludarabine, which has much less side effects than many others. I have developed a rash around the port site, which is very bother-some. The cause is unknown, but Benadryl and a medical ointment is keeping me from climb-ing the walls for now. However, tomorrow, we start to play hard ball. I will continue with the Fludarabine for two more days as well as a dose of Melphalan for both days. The Melphalan is a hard ball drug that is anticipated to make me lose my hair, experience severe nausea, and leave mouth ulcer-type sores from my mouth through-out the rest of the digestive track. So by Tuesday, I should know just how bad the effects will be. I ask you all to pray for God's mercy to be upon this part of the journey in particular.

With the exception of the newly formed rash, things had gone very smoothly. The rash must have been associated with the tubing used for the catheter or local medications, but its source was never found. The constant itching was driving me nuts. I couldn't scratch, when the nurses were around anyway, and I had to be careful not to rub the area and cause infection. So I ground my teeth and prayed extra hard. One thing that did bring relief was when the nurse would wet a washcloth and lay it over the area. The cool damp cloth brought much relief and saved my sanity.

The still waters were about to turn rough. The nurses came in shortly before I was to get Melphalan and, with a big smile, said, "After today and tomorrow, you will no longer want ice in your drinks." The reason was that they had discovered that eating ice before and during the administering of Melphalan reduces the sores in the mouth. I was encouraged to start eating ice, which was plentiful and fresh, and not stop till after the drug had been given. The colder the mouth tissue, the better. For what seemed forever, I munched on ice willing to do whatever I could to lessen the side effects. One cup after another, I crunched and munched. After thirty to forty minutes, the nurses began asking me questions and laughing at my answers. The reason was that I had eaten ice for so long that I could no longer talk plainly. My numb mouth and tongue would slur and mispronounce my words, and we both laughed. I kept eating a never-ending supply of ice.

By midafternoon, I could feel my mouth again and could talk more clearly. It at least seemed that long before my mouth felt anything like normal again. I was able to rest that afternoon and prepare myself for the next round tomorrow.

Cheery and encouraging, the nurses returned the following day with cups of ice. I began to eat. Soon, the chemo was being pushed into my system. And once again, the numbed mouth provided many laughs from mumbled and distorted words. But finally, the chemo treatment was finished.

As the fifth day of the Fludarabine and second day of Melphalan concluded, I was beginning to feel the physical drain and stress they were creating on my body. The well-remembered experiences of a year and a half ago were returning. The nausea was beginning to swell, fatigue was growing, and you could feel your life leaving your body. This time, there were some effects not experienced before. CaringBridge entry:

> Today he had the last day of the chemotherapy. He has begun experiencing the unwanted effects. Foggy thinking, hand tremors, unsteady on his feet, sore mouth and nausea. I (Lauretta) am typing because of the tremors.

I had been warned before having the transplant that I may think I was getting dementia or Alzheimer's, but in time, it would clear up. My memory was getting harder to recall, and my thinking was becoming less focused and rational. I found it very difficult to concentrate on a topic and maintain an ongoing conversation.

As during the first time with chemo, I was hoping the playing of my recorder would not only help pass the time but would bring comfort through playing the hymns of my faith. That was now an impossibility. My hand shook so much I couldn't control holding the recorder and holding my finger over the holes. I couldn't even hold the Bible and read it. Trying to text a message on my phone took so long that the message was no longer relevant once it was completed, seriously. It became my great test of frustration. How would I handle not being able to do the simplest matters of life? I did find one bright spot though, it was in eating. Now I could play in my food and not be chastised for it.

Eating was a frustration in itself. I would make light of it but deep within, it was a painful and dehumanizing experience. Spills were frequent and what started as a fork, more often spoon, full of food often arrived at my lips empty. Fingers were often more effective than utensils. Eating was no longer something enjoyed among others. It was a frustrating exercise I desired to carry out in private. Even sandwiches would wobble as I tried to get them close enough to take a bite out of them. Sometimes, the wobbling would loosen parts of the sandwich that would have to be caught and returned.

EARL J. SPIVEY JR.

One of the secrets I learned was to eat out of a bowl. Bowls have sides you see and plates don't. Trying to catch your meal on a plate can often lead to a chasing about the table. However, when using a bowl, you can chase your food around until you finally get lucky and stab it with your fork or catch it with your fingers against the side of the bowl. I was able to eat the small, square cheesy crackers. They had to be put in a bowl, and I could then corner them so I could grasp them with my fingers. The only problem was that while I went on the attack for one, several others would be tossed out of the bowl in the frantic effort. It really was that bad. It became one of the most difficult side effects to gracefully accept.

As I type this, it is now over 120 days since my transplant. I still have problems typing. My thumb in particular keeps hitting the mouse pad on my laptop and moving my cursor in some unwanted place. My twitching still requires much concentration to hit the keys desired. I frequently make mistakes that frustrate my typing efforts. However, I have come a long way.

I was greatly blessed to have very few mouth sores. I had heard many horror stories of patients with their mouth covered in raw sores. That motivated me to eat ice. I ate it and ate it and ate it some more. The nurses were right. The day following my two Melphalan treatments, I was quiet content to drink my tea without any ice. Slowly, the pleasure of having ice in my drinks returned.

Each day for the next month, the doctors would carefully check my mouth. I had a few sores in the very back of my mouth creating some, though not major, interference with eating. Swallowing was sometimes painful, but I took joy in knowing it was only temporary and in time, the pain would be gone. And before long, it left.

For the next several weeks, eating was one of my less desirable daily activities. I was told the chemo was creating havoc all through my digestive system. There was discomfort in eating and digesting my meals. There was also the out of sorts feeling in my digestive system that told me not to press the issue. It was obvious that my system was in a massive damage control and recovery phase. My choices of food became very selective, and my desire for eating was in a holding pattern until my system invited me to resume eating. I lived on crackers, which I chewed and swallowed very carefully.

A couple of other editable selections were cookies. But with the few sores that I had in my mouth, I didn't want anything hard to chew and digest. I reached back to one of the enjoyments I had had for many years. Chocolate chip cookies, Oreo cookies, and vanilla wafers were three cookies I ate in a preferred way. The whole cookie would be placed into my mouth, and a swallow of milk would follow it. The cookie and milk would sit together in my mouth until the cookie disintegrated. Then with little chewing and little effort in swallowing, the sweet delicious mouthful could be passed on to the awaiting stomach. My sisters kept me in an abundant supply of all of these for the next several weeks. They were my lifeline and my main eating source. I would eat some other foods as well, but these gave me much pleasure, a little nutrition, and very little pain in eating them.

I was surprised to learn that it only took twenty-four hours for the chemo to be gone from my system. Its effect would last much longer and grow in intensity though. That was all the time needed before I could receive the donor stem cells. It was on Tuesday morning, day 0, that the nurses entered with IV bag in hand and said, "Happy birthday, Mr. Spivey."

I jokingly said, "Today, I become my sister's son." In a truer sense, I was to become my sister's twin. Physically and mentally, I was the person I have always been. But genetically, I would now become an extension of my sister.

The IV bag was connected, and the stem cells began entering my body. No weird or cosmic sensations, just an awareness that I was now dead. My blood system that kept me alive for fifty-nine years was destroyed, and I was a dead man still alive. As the stem cells continued flowing down the IV tube and through the pump machine, I was much aware that this dead man was being given a new life. If I lived one week, one year, or one decade, each breath of life was the result of another's gift of life. Each heartbeat would be a testimony of someone's love for my life. Each pleasure and meaningful experience a precious gift undeserved but made possible by becoming the extension of another person's life.

Throughout the time of the continued flowing of stem cells into my veins, I thought of my spiritual new life. I reflected upon my deadness and being given life through Jesus Christ. I was again humbled to think that God looked with kindness on this undeserving soul and brought spiritual life to his dead soul. And through these many years of following Christ, the joys, trials, treasured times, peace, and comfort as well as the moments of special strength were the result of my being an extension of Christ's life. I still remember and give thanks that I have a personal experience that helps me grasp God's love for me in Christ.

It was an emotionally moving day, no doubt. My wife beside me and later my sister, the donor, and her husband would join us. Slowly, the stem cells left the bag and disappeared into my subclavian IV line. I was fortunate in that my arms were both free. Unlike my sister, I could drink and snack if desired. But ice water was still not on my list of beverages. My wife and I watched the disappearing stem cells and quietly wandered through our private thoughts.

That afternoon, my donor sister came over after she finished the stem cell harvesting. We hugged and wept as the second bag, just harvested that day, was being hung on the IV pole. She asked how I was doing, and I said back, "I'm doing fine, but I have the irresistible urge to wear a pair of big blue earbobs." We both laughed. She liked wearing large earrings.

The day passed uneventfully. No medical emergencies or trauma, just an emotionally demanding and tiring day. It was a day of no return. Part of me was gone and now part of someone else would live within me giving me life. It was a day of new beginnings. I was as good as dead. Yet now I have a hope for tomorrow. Would this new life change me? It was a day of spiritual overtones and would they deepen my fellowship with Christ? The tiredness won out, and I finally fell asleep.

Day 1, the first day of my new life, had finally arrived. No fireworks or fanfare. It was just another day in the hospital. I was medically doing well, though well at this point wasn't so good. My numbers were falling, but that was expected. My energy was all but gone and that was normal. My desire to eat was slowly starting to improve. That seemed to be the only positive thing happening at the moment.

Later in the afternoon, I thought I might be able to eat a little something. About the time I ordered my supper, they came in with a syringe of Methotrexate. This was a form of chemo that would be taken about every other week to help hold back any leukemia cells that may have survived the onslaught of the previous chemo treatments. This particular chemo would be used several more times while my baby stem cells were growing. It didn't have any lasting side effects, but nausea was a short term one. Sure enough, by the time my food arrived, I wanted nothing to do with cuisine of any type. My compassionate wife volunteered to remove it so it wouldn't bother me. So she got rid of all of it one bite at a time.

Two days after the transplant, I was able to be discharged. I was surprised that you could leave so soon, but medically you were stable and the side effects I was having did not warrant my staying in the hospital. As I would have to stay within a twenty to thirty-minute drive of the hospital, I could return quickly in the event of worsening conditions, and not returning would be the exception.

The medical coverage I had under Medicaid would cover our housing while required to stay near the hospital. We had worked out the details with the social worker on the transplant team. The day before I was to be discharged, our reservations were made by someone through Medicaid. The name of the hotel was one in which we stayed before while going through the chemo as an outpatient. We double-checked the address and left the hospital for what we thought would be a familiar place.

What we found was a familiar name but an unfamiliar place. The hotel had a newer building, where we had stayed before, and an older hotel building close by it. The older hotel was two stories and all the doors opened to the outside. Whether it was an original building or acquired later by the hotel chain, we never found out. It was a long way from what we were expecting. It became one of the biggest spiritual struggles of my transplant experience.

Lauretta drove around the hotel looking for our room number. When we found it, we both felt deflated. The doorway was directly under a metal stairway leading up to the second floor. Immediately, beside our room was the washroom and dryer vents blowing out heat, moisture, and micro fibers from the drying laundry. I had been warned about bacteria from blowing dust and in the open air, but this was concentrated. We held our breath and went inside.

We stood in the doorway trying to grip emotions for a moment or two and slowly walked in. The room was dark and had a musky smell mixed with air freshener. The doorway was at the foot of the two beds and the narrow walkway led straight ahead to a small table with two chairs. The refrigerator, tiny counter, two burner stove, and small sink were against the back wall. One bed was pushed against the wall and the other against the window air conditioner with a small walkway between them. The floor was covered with a dark carpet that gave much evidence of its having been there for a long time. The bathroom was so cramped that you had to stand beside the toilet to close the door. We sat in the two chairs and were speechless for several moments.

That night and the next day, I wrestled with some spiritual issues. Why did I find this room so disappointing and disheartening? Was it the threat I felt for my physical condition or was it pride? Was God testing my humility and faith in His protection? Was I wanting nice and pleasant conditions because I had too high a regard for myself? My wife and I talked about these matters for some time. I spent much time praying for God to guide me into living humbly for Him and being content with what was given me. But I kept feeling unsafe.

I was on the verge of being physically defenseless. The outside blowing dirt and laundry exhaust was a serious concern. The mold and mildew I feared were in the window air conditioner and carpet left me feeling very vulnerable. The small room and dark atmosphere invited a depressive mood, and we were to be there for about three months. We agreed to talk with the social worker the next morning when we were to return to Hollings.

The social worker came to the infusion room and sat down to talk with us. I shared with her my concerns. She took a deep breath and asked, "Are the sheets clean? Is the floor vacuumed? Do you have clean washcloths and towels?"

"Yes," we replied, "the room seems kept clean, just not sanitary."
She then shared with us that MUSC has little control over the conditions to which the transplant patients return. She shared that many must return to conditions worse than what I was experiencing. It may be that we could ask to be transferred but no promises.

My heart sank, not for my conditions, for the many who, in the most vulnerable phase of their life, would be exposed to unsanitary conditions. Those unsanitary conditions would be responsible for the viral, fungal, and bacterial infections that would take their life. Though hundreds of thousands of dollars were spent on their transplant and more again on treating their avoidable illnesses, the hospital had to discharge them to conditions they knew were potential death traps. Surely, something can be done to stop this!

We went back to our room more heavyhearted than when we left. We wondered if we were to stay or find some way into a better condition. We decided to take the social worker's advice and ask for a room reassignment. If it worked, great. If not, I would commit myself to be content in whatever situation in which I found myself following the Apostle Paul's example. My wife made several phone calls checking into the possibility of a room reassignment. The manager was fine with it and willing to help. The insurance representative following our case said it would depend on the decision of the Medicaid representative managing room assignments. Her response was our last call.

Weeks earlier, we had stayed in the home of a couple in the Mt. Pleasant area. We had a very special time of talking and spiritual sharing while staying with them. Their unused bedrooms on the second floor were being used to house travelers for some extra cash. The time with them made a lasting link between us and a genuine concern over my condition. They had encouraged us to stay with them during the time of my recovery, but I just felt uneasy moving into someone's home I haven't known very long. They also had commitments for people to stay during this time as well. Therefore, we decided to go with Medicaid and stay in a hotel.

I struggled in prayer over our situation. While my wife was talking with the Medicaid representative who was saying that room assignments were final and nothing else could be done, I was praying. "Lord, if you want us to stay with the couple we met several weeks ago, have one of them call and invite us to go there." That was highly unlikely due to a scheduled stay over for that night. As my wife hung up the phone and shared the heartbreaking conclusion, her text message notification sounded. She opened the text message, and tears came to her eyes. It simply said, "Come now…the guest will not be coming due to sickness." I began to weep as well and shared with her that the invitation was the sign I was asking God to send. Another work of divine grace abundantly placed upon us.

My wife packed up what little things we had brought in and made the arrangements to move. The new location provided comfort, space, and excellent sanitary conditions. After all, our host was a nurse. It was in much peace that I now lay in a cheerful environment feeling free of medical fears.

I was still falling to the bottom. My energy was continuing to waste away. My digestive efforts had to be carefully guarded and any new items on the menu gently tried. Most anything eaten was soft in texture. My swallowing was sore and painful, but I continued to be grateful it wasn't worse. An old favorite was helpful, even though my portions were now quite small.

For several years, my grandfather was bedridden and unable to get up. He was not able to chew much of anything due to progressing Parkinson's disease, so my grandmother knew one item he enjoyed was grits over an egg fried easy over. The grits were placed on top of the egg, and then the two were mixed together. The soft egg yolk gave more moisture while the soft white was cut into small pieces. This required little chewing and was nutritious.

I, too, came to enjoy the dish, especially with yellow grits. With the difficulty of chewing and swallowing, this would be a good meal to eat, and it was. I tried milkshakes but found they were too something or other for my digestion as they didn't set too well, but the cookies with a little milk or water were fine.

The weekend was now here, and the children were on their way. My uncle brought them, and we were able to be together, sort of, again. My daughter wanted to stay glued to the TV in the one bedroom while my son was enjoying the fast internet connection in the other bedroom. But we were in the same place and could at least see one another in transit from time to time.

I was able to spend some time with my uncle too. He was my father's youngest brother and had been home some during my grammar school days. He had worked on the farm and was a positive role model for me. He had come up from his home in Florida to stay with my children so Lauretta could be by my side. He had stayed once before during my initial diagnosis and hospital stay. It was good to be together again and renew our relationship.

A dear friend for many years came that morning as well. He and I camped the rivers of my home area and shared many struggles together. We were both pastors with a commitment to lead others in going beyond nominal religious experiences and into a life-changing relationship with Christ. We enjoyed being together, and I was glad that I felt well enough to enjoy the company of my uncle and best friend.

The two of them left that afternoon, and it was me and my family together again. We enjoyed the short time we had before my wife, and the children would return home. We had planned to do things a little differently this time.

When I was in the hospital the first time, my wife stayed by my side almost the whole time. She wanted to be with me and help care for me as she knew my medical situation and my need for someone else to help. We had various family members and friends to stay with the children who were at that time twelve and thirteen. It went well for the most part, but preacher's kids will be preacher's kids. This time, we thought it would be better for them emotionally for sure for Lauretta to be at home and maintain household routines and parental guidance. They were now fourteen and fifteen.

Sunday afternoon, my youngest sister came to be with me for the week, and Lauretta and the children returned home. I was going through the worst time and would soon start improving. My condition seemed to be leveling off and hopefully, I wouldn't be experiencing any more serious side effects. We said our good-byes and waved them off.

The biggest challenge of staying with me was to keep track of my medications and temperature. A printed guide was prepared for us so giving me my medications was as simple as checking off a list. The time, medication and amount were noted with a box to check each time the medication was taken. I couldn't be trusted because during a bad thinking moment, I, in confusion, might take too much or skip a medicine. So my sister guarded the dispensary and every four to six hours stuck a thermometer in my mouth. I had several temperature spikes to about ninety-nine, but they would always drop back down. The take action mark was 100.5. If I reached a fever that high, then call the doctor on the way to the hospital. If it was around one hundred, call and await a decision.

The next several days were mostly routine. Wake up, take my thyroid med one hour before eating. Next, take the remainder of my meds with something to eat if I could. The meds had to be taken regardless. Sometimes, I would fall back to sleep and sometimes sit up in a chair. About lunchtime, I would try to eat something if nothing more than softened cookies. I had one or two meds that needed to be taken in early afternoon as well. Then it would be time to talk, sit up, or take a nap if I wasn't feeling well. At suppertime, I would try to eat something again. It may be grits and egg, oatmeal, apple sauce or anything I thought my digestive system would accept. Then I relaxed until med time again, around 8:00 p.m. In between was the temperature checking and familiar questions, "Are you feeling okay? Any pain anywhere? Want something to eat or drink?" and a few others from time to time.

I found myself going through one of the oldest medical mysteries that is still not resolved. "Why do patients get worse in the late afternoon and evenings?" It is witnessed so many times but still no explanation for the condition. For me, it was feeling worse and running a low-grade fever. By Monday, I would start running a fever about three to four in the afternoon, and it would climb until about nine at night. Then, as mysteriously as it appeared, it would fade away. We watched it closely, but since it didn't rise above one hundred degrees, we didn't call the doctor on call.

Wednesday afternoon, the fever was back again. Only this time, it kept rising to a hundred degrees. My sister called in as instructed and the doctor said, "Bring him on in, and we will check to be sure nothing serious is happening." And off to the hospital we went.

I was taken into the emergency room and placed in a separate out of the way room. They were extra careful to help me avoid any contact with viruses or bacteria brought in by other patients. This would require the familiar stick in the arm to check for infection. The nurse did all the work ordered and called the cancer doctor on call. By now, my fever was starting to drop again. I was feeling a little better.

The cancer doctor soon came in and talked with me. She went over the findings and decided to admit me back into the cancer ward to be sure nothing serious was developing. It was not unexpected. I had been told by nurses and doctors that recovery would be a roller-coaster ride. Very few patients do not have to return to the hospital and stay to fight off infections. It was just part of the critical immune system weakness. I was taken to a familiar place and hoped that my stay would be a short one. My hope was to be a false hope.

Once in the room out came the IV pole and a yellowish bag of platelets. Before that bag was finished, two different antibiotics were added. The doctors know the danger of even the smallest infection at this critical phase of my recovery. So the doctor did just as they had said earlier, "We're gonna bring out the big guns now and stop whatever is attacking." For the next couple of days, it was an all-out assault against the enemy even though the enemy wasn't identified.

My sister was to stay till Saturday so now she made herself as comfortable as possible and remained by my side day and night. I had to be careful what I said because if she heard me say, "I think I would like..." or "You know _____ would be good," she would do all she could to see that I had it. And usually, it would be in abundance. She was passionate about giving her brother the best care he could get. My room was well stocked with crackers and cookies ready for my consumption.

My sister, many would say, is a very religious person. But she and I both knew that there is a huge difference between being religious and spiritual. As the apostle Paul noted, we can observe the letter of the law in detail and yet not live the intent of the law. We both knew that Christianity was a relationship we had with Christ and not a meeting of particular religious requirements. We talked of our faith and journey with Christ. Because I could not hold the Bible and read, she would read my daily devotional book for me each night before I went to sleep. Throughout the weeks, those staying with me did the same.

I had been back in the hospital just a day or two, but I was tired and struggling. The side effects were weighing heavy on me. The recognition that my visit was not to be a quick fix me up and send me home visit was hard to accept. My inability to eat and the all-round discomforts were weights I was finding difficult to carry. It was about 6:00 a.m. I had just taken my first round of meds and was wide awake. My sister was awake too and sat up to talk "You okay?"

"Yes, I'm okay. I want you to help me do something."

"All right, what is it?"

"I want you to help me get down on my knees and spend some time in prayer."

She was very agreeable, of course. I knew that if I made it down on my knees, I would have a very difficult time getting up. I also knew that this was my best time of the day to spend some time in the garden of prayer. We kneeled together and for about forty-five minutes poured out our hearts in prayer. It was a refreshing time for me and helped me in carrying the weights that seemed to be collecting on me. And more weights began clinging.

It was Saturday and my sister was to leave, and my wife and children to come for the weekend. This Sunday would be Easter, and I would still be in the hospital. I was developing a pain in my right shoulder and a cold feeling in my hand. An ultrasound was taken, and I had a nonserious blood clot. It would eventually go away by itself. I would have another dose of Methotrexate, and that would ruin my afternoon and evening. I was already nauseated and that only made it worse. I also noticed that my hair was starting to fall out. Other than that, I was just completely miserable.

As my wife and children left, I was feeling worse. The old fever was returning, and I could feel myself losing altitude rapidly. Here is what I dictated to my sister to put on CaringBridge.

> Let us praise the Lord for His loving-kindness endures forever. Earl J., by the hand of my sister. Once more, God has touched me with his healing hand. Yesterday was the lowest of days. Were it not for a visit from my two sisters and brother-in-law, it would have been most difficult to endure. I had dizziness, heaviness in chest, nausea, and difficulty breathing. Low enough to contemplate final arrangements. But God showed great mercy over the night. I awoke with no heaviness of chest and a new freedom to breathe. No nausea and ready for something to eat and drink. Doctors affirm that the stem cells are producing white blood cells and platelets so the road to recovery has begun. The chest X-ray showed no problems but a little fluid in one lung. So back to eating, exercising, and working toward recovery. So we give praise to God for His kindness and hand of mercy. Blessings upon you all.

It was a tough way to start the week but a great time to feel God's touch. Relief seemed to have finally come. The return of hope brought much joy to me. Now, it appeared that I was finally climbing up and not sliding further down the darkened pit.

The next couple of days seemed to be days of hope and encouragement. My white blood cells were starting to climb. My platelet count was rising as well. Both were indicators of bone marrow production. We just hope it is from the new cells and not any leftover old cells.

My sister and I enjoyed a lot of laughs and reviewing of old stories. She worked hard to see that I was as comfortable as possible.

She also encouraged me to eat and drink for my health. My wife was to return later in the week so my sister could return home.

Thursday, the alarm bells began to sound. Although my blood numbers were coming up, my breathing was growing harder by the hour. The doctors knew I had some water around my lungs and were trying to remove it with Lasix. The Lasix didn't seem to be getting rid of the fluid. So the lung doctors were called in. They found inflammation in my lungs but were unable to determine what was causing it. In consultation with the cancer doctors, they thought it might be the results of the rapid rise in my white blood count.

With the difficulty in breathing, my heart was feeling the stress. It began to show sign of weakening. The old enemy—atrial fibrillation—was returning. The techs checked my blood pressure and heart rate to discover a heart rate of nearly two hundred. That brought me lots of attention. It also brought me the annoying monitor to be worn around my neck again.

The daily blood test revealed that my creatinine level was rising. The creatinine numbers reveal the condition of your kidneys. If they are working well, your creatinine level will be low. But if you are flirting with kidney failure, your level will rise. Mine had started to rise. So in came the kidney doctors to help keep me out of kidney failure.

It seemed the only doctors that hadn't been called in were the psychiatrists. I was beginning to think I might need them too. The world was suddenly crashing down on me. By Saturday, I was started on oxygen again, and my day was spent entertaining doctors. My wife was watching everything closely and talking in detail with the doctors. I was just there.

As my wife returned home and my brother-in-law took over for the week, my ship was taking on water. The doctors were in a mad scramble to get a proper diagnosis of my problems and respond to alleviate my struggle. As the week slowly passed, X-rays and tests were done to diagnose what was happening. Was it the chemo, my heart, my lungs or all of the above? Whatever it was, I was getting worse and nothing seemed to stop it.

My eating had decreased while my oxygen was increased. I was building up fluid and not getting rid of it. I was too exhausted to walk so I mostly lay helpless to fight off what was destroying me. My brother-in-law stood by me and did all he could to help me. Day after day, I grew weaker, and the doctors drew no closer to solving the problem.

Up went the oxygen. Up went the creatinine. The heart rate fluctuated and kept the nurses in suspense. Up came the white blood cells, platelets, and immune system. But we all wondered if the new cells were the problem. The inflammation expanded, and nothing was halting its advance. And day after day, I wondered if I had passed the point of no return. I was slowly coming apart, and I had no power to stop my disintegrating health.

My wife returned for the weekend alone. It was better that way. I was all but gone, and it would have been hard for the children to stay in the room and watch me weakened and the doctors struggling for a way to help. The weekend decreased the number of doctors coming in each day, but someone from the four areas came by each day.

I was now entering my third week in the hospital. I came in with a fever, and it had turned into a major medical situation. It was not uncommon. Time and again, the nurses stood by watching someone who had been doing so well just a week or so before falling apart. They could do all they were trained to do. They could carefully follow the doctor's orders. They could be encouraging and pleasant with the patients and still the patient gets worse and worse until death engulfs them. Maybe that is why so few older nurses are on that floor. Most of the nurses are young and just starting in their career. Burnout can come quickly when the survival rate is low.

By Saturday night, my oxygen was as high as it could go. I had gone from the familiar tube under your nose to what they called the maximizer. I had reached the limit. My lungs were inflamed, and nothing was known to help it. My kidneys were about to quit, and my liver was showing signs of stress. My heart was erratic and unpredictable. And I was losing my will to fight. My heart doctor was trying to cheer me on, but I wasn't finding much strength for fighting.

Monday was a day of painful reality. One by one, my doctors entered my room to give me their final evaluations and assessments.

The kidney doctors said my kidneys were on the verge of not working, and they had no way to prevent it. If they improved, it would not be as a result of their efforts to help.

The heart doctors said that my heart was stressed and about to give out. If I could hold on a little longer, it may be able to regain its strength.

The lung doctors told me that the fluid around my lungs was too much for the medications to remove. I was not able to stand the procedure for drawing the fluid off and if they did, it would just return. The inflammation was getting close to covering my entire lungs. They had nothing else they could do. If I grew any worse, all they could do was to move me to ICU and put me on a breathing machine. It was now up to my body to heal itself.

My cancer doctors only said they were out of options and that they hoped and prayed that my body could somehow overcome the many medical problems. They encouraged me to hold on and not give up.

I struggled through the night to keep breathing and not go to ICU. I began to feel the weight was too great to remove. I had peace in saying good-bye to this world. I was tired of the fighting. I was starting to feel homesick for Christ's promise to His followers, an eternal life without the suffering and sorrows of this world.

By Tuesday morning, my condition was no better. I felt the medical opposition was more than I could defeat. I felt overwhelmed by the many physical complications that were like lead weights on a weary swimmer. I accepted that death was now close, and I could not resist it any longer. I prayed for God to give me peace in the transition and courage to rest in Him. Then I told my wife.

"Lauretta," I said softly.

"What is it?" she said in response.

"I'm not going home with you. I think I've gone as far as I can. Here is what I want done."

For the next thirty minutes, I shared with her how my funeral was to be conducted and what was to be done with my body. We both choked on the tears and lump in our throats but knew denying the inevitable was useless. We were grateful for the spiritual hope we shared and held tightly the promise of God's acceptance for all who trusted in His Son.

I lay back in peace accepting whatever was to come. The doctors came by one after another and affirmed that no change was occurring that offered any hope for recovery. Everyone was standing by hoping I would not get any worse but feeling that I wasn't going to get any better. I listened with little response. I fought for each breath while I awaited the great transition.

My wife was to go home that day and my dear friend Denley was to stay with me for a couple of days. I encouraged my wife to go home and be with the children. She said what we thought might well be the last good-bye and affirmed her love for me. Then she left Denley and me to wait in the comfort of God's grace.

What happened next no one expected, certainly not me. Here is how my wife described it:

> I was to come home that day but wasn't sure about leaving. A friend was to come and spend the night. We decided I would come on home. Denley arrived in the afternoon. He called me that night and said something to the effect. "If I hadn't seen it for myself, I wouldn't have believed it. Sorry you missed it." He told me he could see Earl J improving every hour. Wednesday morning proved Earl J doing a lot better and the improvement continues. He sounds great. All praise goes to God. And a huge thanks for all of your prayers. I texted Earl J's sisters today that we had "cast our cares on Him" (Jesus Christ), 1 Peter 5:7. God took care of the rest according to His plans and will; and to His glory. Children and I will be traveling down tomorrow. Can't wait to see him.

It had to be God's miraculous touch upon my life. The doctors were admittedly no longer to give help. I was tired and ready for the great transformation. No one showed hope of my overcoming. But "more than conquerors" I became. It wasn't in my strength. It was something beyond me. Some will say it was a medical fluke. Some will pass it off as a mystery. I and many others acknowledge it as a miracle, a gift placed upon me. Each hour, I could feel strength returning. Hope had returned and the old mule spirit was being rebirthed. By supper, it was clear that I was not going to die. I was instead going to experience a power beyond myself to return to the land of the living.

One by one, I began to take the steps on the long stairway that would lead me up from the pit of earthly hopelessness. I could feel my breathing change. I could almost take a deep breath again. The oxygen was still all the way up, but my sensations told me improvement had begun.

> Since Tuesday, the Lord has continued to bless Earl J with improvement. He said to a sister, "I'm climbing out of the well". He wanted to walk this morning without O2, nurses were agreeable. His O2 saturation dropped low once but picked back up after a brief rest. He has not used the oxygen all day and walked a second time without any problem.

The above was written on the following Sunday. From Wednesday onward, daily progress was made, cutting back on the oxygen little by little. A new energy and commitment to climb out of the well I felt I was in. The nurses were excited to see me getting better and defying the claims of death. The doctors rejoiced to see that I hadn't become another patient lost in their attempts to help. They may credit it to luck, physical stamina, or anything else, but several knew that God stopped me from certain death and had given me new life. From eating to getting out of bed, from a renewed spirit to a mule-like determination, I had experienced a complete turn-around, and the hospital staff was watching. They had given up. I had surrendered. And then God revealed His power. A miracle that drew the attention and praise of so many in the hospital and in many churches as well! Praise the Lord!

Hope had returned and the sun was now rising instead of setting. One by one, the groups of doctors were releasing me due to the improvement of my condition. The only lasting doctors were the heart and cancer doctors. With their kind favor, I was released just one week from the day I was ready to enter the eternal world. Unlike the discharge when diagnosed, I now left with life swelling within and determination to return to the work left for the time of transplant. I couldn't go far, but at least, I was out of the hospital. The hotel room was a wonderful change from the bed, instruments, nursing rounds, and 4:00 a.m. weigh-in.

For the first few weeks, I was to report three times a week to the cancer center. The usual blood work and visit with a doctor or nurse practitioner filled the morning. At first, I was required to be at the cancer center by 7:30 a.m. That was because of the weakness of my immune system. They would have the more recent transplant patients come in early so they would be less exposed to the potential viruses, bacteria, etc., that were brought in by the other patients and those accompanying them. On the weekend, the cancer center was closed, and a mini-center was located on the cancer floor of the hospital. They could do most everything done at the cancer center on Saturday and Sunday.

We would leave the hotel early and make our way to either the cancer center or hospital. They would draw a number of vials of blood and once the tests results were available on their computer, they determined if I needed blood, platelets, magnesium, or anything else before being released to go home. Other patients would be in the room and often, conversations were made among various patients and caregivers. Unless I needed an infusion, I would be able to return home by midmorning. If I needed an infusion, it would be lunchtime or after before leaving. We always came with a snack and meds, not knowing if the visit would be short or long. But long was the norm for the next several weeks.

With the help of a walker, I was able to move about. I had to go slow and inclines were particularly troublesome until my strength increased. But with determination and the joy of being almost free again, I was ready to move and rejoice in my new freedom. The long walk to the room was exhausting, but it was better than having to ride in a wheelchair. I soon began to exercise by walking up and down the hallway on the days I didn't go to the clinic. On those days, I would get enough exercise. And day by day, I could tell that my strength was slowly returning. Moving about was getting easier, and I could even take a shower by myself. I could stand up to brush my teeth. I soon was able to walk to the bathroom by using the wall or furniture to help me remain steady and be free of the walker. Slowly, I felt like I was coming alive again.

The weeks passed slowly. The doctors emphasized to keep things boring. What they meant was no fevers, mysterious sicknesses, or GvHD (graft versus host disease). By God's grace, no fevers came, no illnesses to battle, and not even any sign of rejection by the new blood system now inhabiting my body. But boredom was the new struggle.

I was able to do a little reading but not much. The same was with the computer. I still shook too much to do any serious work on the keyboard. I did punch out several posts on the CaringBridge site, but with much difficulty. I was getting strong enough to be able to go out and eat and grew excited to leave the hotel room. I was still too weak to do any sightseeing and honestly wasn't much interested. For the next few weeks, we remained in the hotel. Regular trips to the cancer clinic, outings for lunch and supper, and finally back to church.

Years before, I was in a pastoral support group with a pastor from Georgetown. He moved to Mt. Pleasant after a year or so of our time together. Now that I was out of the hospital and able to be around a crowd sparing and cautiously, I wanted to hear him preach and worship at the church he pastored. After a couple of weeks, the weekend trips to the clinic in the hospital were dropped, and Sunday's were free for me to attend worship. My wife, children, and I would attend each Sunday for the next several weeks. My family usually came down for the weekend as school was still in session and worship was part of our Sunday routine whether I was the pastor or not.

I would get out as close to the door as possible. My two children, both teenagers, would help me making sure I didn't stumble and fall with the walker. I was wearing a mask, of course, and flannel jacket even though it was now June. I am writing this in July and still wear a jacket in any air-conditioned place. Our thermostat is set at seventy-three degrees. My wife thinks it is hot, but I sit close by in my jacket. At night, I use several covers to keep me warm. And I think it is delightful to go somewhere on these hot July days because I get to get in the car warmed by the sun and just soak-in the heat. It is just part of the process. Whether blood thinners or side effect, this is the first summer that the heat is fine with me.

I enjoyed being back in a community worship service again. The people were nice and accepting of my mask. I thought I might be searched or escorted by a security guard, but all seemed to recognize I had a medical condition and welcomed me to worship with them. It was difficult to stand and sometimes, I had to remain seated. Singing was a love I had been denied for a long time. To whisper the words of the praise songs or hymns was all I could do. I didn't have enough breath to sing, but I still had a spirit with which to give thanks and praise. And I now had strength to return to the place of worship and honor the God who extended my life.

Music and singing, in particular, was always an important part of my life. My mother was a gifted vocalist and sang for many occasions as well as the church choir. My father could hold the bass line pretty well also. My sisters and I all grew up with piano lessons and much encouragement to participate in musical experiences. I sang in the youth choir and then adult choir at church while going to college. When away at college, I sang in the college choir and a vocal team that sang for various churches on the weekend.

I had learned to sing parts in my older youth years and had a voice high enough to sing tenor. Tenor or bass were parts I would sing to add more harmony to the melody. Once my heart was surrendered to Christ during my first year of college, my singing became my avenue of worship and experiencing God's delight in me, His child. As a pastor, I had led the choir, praise team, and other special musical groups throughout the years.

After my first two rounds of chemo and then throughout the experimental drug taken for the following year and a half, my singing was very limited. At first, I was unable to sing due to my lack of breath. As my lungs slowly improved, I was able to croak out a line or two before stopping to regain my breath.

One of the most disappointing losses leukemia has brought to me has been singing. Throughout my waiting for the transplant and now my recovery following transplant, singing tenor is gone. Somehow my vocal cords have changed and my singing is only the bass part, or if I sing the melody line, I must sing it in the low octave. My son sometimes asked me when I was talking, "Dad, why are you using your dark voice?" Sometimes, my talking was much lower. Now I sing in the lower octave the hymns and songs of my faith. Once in a while, I'll sing bass in the hymn's four-part harmony. I've not dared to return to the choir though I often watch and listen missing greatly the joy of singing so others can experience joy in their faith.

Perhaps one day, singing will return. For now, solos and the beautiful harmony of the tenor voice will be absent in my life. I can still sing and rejoice through music. One of my great joys is missing, but my joy of listening with the heart remains. So I'll sing whatever part and in whatever octave my vocal cords will allow.

As my digestive system began healing from the damages of the chemo, my ability to eat grew. That was good as I was being put on a heavy dosage of Prednisone to fight the inflammation in my lungs. And everybody knows Prednisone makes hunger a major part of life. I ate like a horse. Though I had to watch what I ate and how much I ate, I wanted to eat all the time. I had by then moved far enough past the transplant that my system was recovering. Each meal became a test of my body's ability to eat, digest, and not rebel at my overdose of food. It wasn't until I was weaned off the Prednisone that my eating was slowed and the continual craving for something to eat left.

Even with all my eating, my weight only grew minutely. Actually, my body was working overtime to heal what the chemo had damaged. With the intensive use of energy, it wanted overtime nutrition. I was encouraged to graze on the calories and gobble up the proteins. So this was the closest I have come to a license to sin. It was my one freedom during the medical restraints and restrictions. Day after day, I broadened my selections and enjoyed eating whenever and whatever—that is, as much as my stomach and intestines would allow.

After a week in the hotel, we were able to return to the comforts of the couple's home where we were staying before. They had a week of prior commitments reserving the rooms. Once fulfilled, we were able to return. Lauretta stayed with me for a couple of weeks, partly due to it being easier to get someone to stay with our children than with me. I probably was more trouble. We returned to the clinic three times weekly. My head doctor decided to put me back on the experimental drug for a few months as extra insurance in holding back and eliminating any leftover leukemia cells. That meant another stay in the hospital.

Though short, this was emotionally a very difficult stay in the hospital. I had been on Tikosyn for my heart since the cardioversion in late January. When I was being readied for the transplant, they stopped the Tikosyn due to feared interactions with the differing drugs used during the transplant. Now that I was improving, they didn't want my heart relapsing into atrial fibrillation due to added stress. As shared earlier, the drug Tikosyn had to be started in the hospital where my heart could be observed twenty-four hours a day. I tried to prepare for returning to the hospital but dreaded the necessity.

Into the hospital I went and SNAFU, situation normal all fouled up, returned all over again. I checked in on Friday ready for a "hit it and git gone" stay. This would be my fourth stay in the hospital. Each time I went in, I came out much weaker and further behind physically. I had just finally been given a new hope for life, and I feared the hospital stay would lead to further physical deterioration. Mentally, I feared another crumbling of my health. I prayed for strength and peace to stay and go through the necessary medical process.

As you can imagine, my cardiologist was frustrated. He had worked with me to get my heart in its regular rhythm after my diagnosis. When my post hospital chemo failed, the medication had to be stopped due to the experimental drug. When I went back into atrial fibrillation while on the study drug, he again returned my heart to a normal rhythm with cardioversion and another drug. Shortly thereafter, the transplant team told him that Tikosyn was not compatible with the treatment drugs. As a result, we had to stop all heart-regulating drugs and go on prayer and hopes for no serious heart interruptions. Now, after all that, he was asked to restart me on Tikosyn in preparation for the added stress the experimental would bring.

Once in the hospital, the cardiologist on rounds was actually over my case. He and his team evaluated my condition and long list of medications and found one not compatible with Tikosyn. It was stopped, not being a priority medication. Saturday morning, the dark visitor returned to my room.

The team was still evaluating the many interactions between Tikosyn and my other medications. The tech came in as usual to get my stats. She took my stats twice and called for the EKG machine. Atrial fibrillation was back. In comes the nurses, in comes the doctors; back in my bed I go with orders to stay there. I still could not tell I was in atrial fibrillation, but the medical staff knew it and acted decisively to respond to it.

Shortly, my heart jumped back into its normal rhythm. As a result, the intensity of the situation decreased, but the nurses were now on high alert. *So much for Tikosyn today!* I thought. The old familiar nightmare appeared to be returning.

My frustration was rising quickly. By Saturday afternoon, I was still in the hospital and yet to have any idea when I would take the first dose. Delays, contemplations, and emotional disappointment fell hard. I wanted to go AWOL (absent without leave). I was finally starting to regain what was lost, and now it seemed that if I stayed in the hospital, it would all be lost again. I was fighting hard to maintain a pleasant disposition with the nurses and doctors. They could tell that I was growing anxious and troubled. The doctor was a very personable man. He would sit and talk, and I knew he was serious about doing what was best for my health. It was just that everything within me was screaming to run. But God gives grace for us to withstand the pressures that push us. Running was not an option, only continued obedience and trust.

Saturday afternoon, the doctor on call came to assure me that the first dosage would be started the next morning. He shared how they were carefully evaluating my medications and wanted to be sure the interactions would not be harmful. It helped much to talk with the doctor and hear of his concerns and cautious actions. I eagerly awaited the first pill. Sunday morning, it came and finally, I felt like progress was being made.

Since I was in the heart unit, my diet was more restricted. Several of the choices that I was using before were now off limits. Add to that my level of frustration and my appetite was way down. All I wanted was to get out of the hospital and back to the home where I was staying. There I could regain my positive focus and prepare myself for going home. My heart stayed in its normal rhythm, and the taking of the heart medications seemed to be going well. Sunday passed without any excitement, and Monday proved to be smooth and without any more medical interruptions.

Tuesday came and all was looking well. The doctor and team of students made the morning rounds and said everything was going well. So there was revived hope in leaving the hospital soon. It was after lunch that the doctor came in by himself. Not on his rounds, no students, unexpected. *This isn't good*, I thought. He had a solemn tone when he spoke.

"Mr. Spivey, we are going to stop the Tikosyn."

I held my breath wondering just what he was about to say. I didn't feel medically troubled. I didn't think there were any problems right now. I leaned forward and listened. My wife was leaning with me.

"Our research has revealed that the Tikosyn in combination with your study drug could be lethal. So we are going to stop it."

My first thought was, *Then what comes next and how much longer will I have to stay in the hospital?* So I asked.

He shared with me that there were no further options. I would have to go without a regulating medication and hope for the best. He reaffirmed that since I did not know when I went into atrial fibrillation, I could live years with it if it came back and my heart didn't return to its normal rhythm. Also, once the experimental drug was discontinued, I could go back on one of the medications then. My personal cardiologist would decide then. As for the hospital stay, they would continue to do an EKG that night and watch me until morning and if all was good, I could be discharged tomorrow. I prayed for all to be good until I fell asleep.

On Wednesday morning, I awoke to find all was well. During his daily rounds, the doctor gave the order to discharge me. Once the medications were all in order, I would be free to leave. About lunchtime, we left the hospital and returned to the home where I once more found comfort and renewed hope.

I was now ten pounds less than when I entered the hospital. I was still using the walker because my legs were just too weak. I had an appointment to return to the clinic, and I prayed that would be as close to the hospital as I would have to go. Now I could get food to build up my strength. Now I could move about without constant observation and fear of a nurse's detecting something wrong. Though my wife kept a close eye, only the significant medical issues would be addressed. I was finally free again.

Back at the home in Mt. Pleasant, my wife remained by my side while family members kept watch over our children. She worked hard to shuffle me back and forth to the clinic. I had to prepare for the experimental drug by taking another thorough eye exam, and I had the necessary bone marrow biopsy before I left the hospital. Now it was time to go back on the study drug. But the sun was shining brightly as my health was beginning to return. CaringBridge entry:

> From Earl: Yesterday and today were most wonderful days. My progress is going well and my system is adjusting to the experimental drug I started on again last week. The doctors have been very cautious about its effect upon my heart. So every day, I go back to the clinic to take an EKG and blood test. Though feeling sorry for my spending so much time at the clinic, they felt it necessary to closely monitor my weakened heart. So back and forth we went day after day.

At least it gave us something to do each morning. I was glad to be in the couple's house but with limited abilities, boredom grew. I began to watch TV, which I haven't done in many years. I tried to watch a few baseball games and couldn't regain my enjoyment for sports from the many years earlier. I did enjoy documentaries on the History channel and liked several programs on the Discovery and Animal Planet channels. Often, I would settle for an afternoon nap and give my body some rest.

It was during this week that one of the biggest moments of my journey arrived. CaringBridge entry:

> Yesterday, we were told that test results indicate that none, that is "not nary a one," of my old blood cells were detected, only the blood cells coming from my new stem cells. So the old Earl Jackson Spivey Jr. is dead and the new one lives. I am sure that test will be repeated later, but as God has been so good to me, I trust none of the old leukemia-laced cells will be found. Praise the Lord. Today, we returned with the encouraging news that my heart rate seemed steady, and my magnesium level was still up where they wanted it. So the doctor's assistant informed us that she, the doctor, and others discussed it and that I was not to return until Monday. Wow! I get the whole weekend off.

It was time for shouting and dancing. The first real mark of my being cleansed from leukemia was shown. It wasn't a declaration of healing, but it was much more than hope and certainly a time to celebrate. The celebration would come that weekend when my brother-in-law came. He wanted to get away to a local hotel since relatives had come to stay with the couple. That would keep us from disturbing them and give us time to get away and celebrate God's blessings.

Another significant step had been taken that week. It had not taken place since leaving the hospital after my transplant now some two month ago. CaringBridge entry:

> Thanks to your prayers I am feeling well and today decided to go unassisted. I'm talking about the walker. I left it on purpose when going to the clinic this morning and did well. I felt a little like a kid's first ride without training wheels but all went well.

It was a wonderful week of physical advancements. Hope was shining brightly and joyful anticipations of the future were returning. So Friday after lunch, my brother-in-law arrived, and we prepared to celebrate.

We went to an upscale hotel he was familiar with through the bank where he worked. We settled in the room and began making arrangement for eating. Most days, I could eat well and once in a while, I just had a day I didn't feel like eating, usually due to nausea. We had a big supper and returned to the room to sleep it off.

Saturday, we had a big breakfast. Some close friends came by with all sorts of goodies and an enjoyable time of sharing together. I wasn't up for much at lunch so we watched a movie and planned for a big meal for supper. We enjoyed the meal, although I ate cautiously and paid close attention to my digestive system.

Sunday, we both wanted to be in worship, and I had a lot for which to give thanks and celebrate. We enjoyed our breakfast and made our way to the worship service. Though I couldn't sing much, I rejoiced and whispered my thanksgiving to the God who had brought me through this valley filled with death. I celebrated His goodness to me by guiding the doctors to discover the lethal potential of the medication I was supposed to have taken. I thanked God for His comfort, presence, and provisions to my family throughout this difficult journey. And then with a refreshed spirit, we left to enjoy one last meal together before his returning home.

After we ate, he took me back to the home in Mt. Pleasant and settled me back into my room. I had encouraged Lauretta to just wait and return the next morning in time to take me to the clinic. I was doing well except for a little more difficulty in breathing and would be fine by myself until she arrived. CaringBridge entry:

> Earl J says, "The horse has three legs and a wagon wheel wobbles." I say it is just a bump in the road. I drove down yesterday morning to take him to the clinic. His face looked puffy to me and the physician's assistant noticed it also. When weighed, he had gained 10 pounds in five days. They were glad it was caught early but to make sure it didn't get worse, he was admitted to the hospital for "a few days". This way, they can tackle it faster and halt continued damage to his body.

It must have been a bigger weekend than I thought. The weight gain was fluid around my heart and lungs. That is why my breathing began feeling more difficult. Be sure your sins will find you out. But the weekend was a wonderful timeout from the routine and a day or two in the hospital, and a heavy dose of Lasix wasn't too high a price to pay.

It was back to the heart floor that I went and in came the Lasix. Unlike the other stays, this one was smooth and quick. The Lasix drew off eight pounds of fluid by nightfall. My heart was beating in its regular rhythm, and all seemed to be going well. The next day, the doctors said I was doing well and should be able to be discharged the following day.

It was on Monday that we learned that the college age children of the home where I had been staying had to return for the summer to their mother's home. That meant we would no longer be able to stay there. The couple felt bad, but we assured them they had been a blessing and a comfort to us, and we understood the sudden change of plans. Surprises are part of life.

I still had at least a month to go before being able to return home. My wife and I talked about what we would do as the cost of a hotel room for that period of time was more than we could afford. I suggested that we contact the social worker to see if Medicaid would still provide us with a room since we declined the first one. So Tuesday, I contacted the social worker, and she investigated it. Medicaid would once again provide lodging until I was free to return home. Once again, we whispered a prayer of thanks and humble gratitude for God's providing us a place at no cost to us. And this time, it would be at a much nicer and sanitary hotel. A comfortable place to be bored!

My dear friend returned for another week of duty. The last several weeks proved difficult to get anyone to be here with me so my wife was working with family and friends to see that the children had rides to school and back and someone to stay with them at night. I had begun feeling better so I encouraged her to leave me for a day and be home with the children. It was difficult on her to travel back and forth, a two-and-a-half-hour drive, but with my appointments being stretched to several days apart, it was workable.

My friend came prepared to cook a camp-style meal as he and I spent many days camping together. He came to find me in the hospital and though I would be discharged a couple of days later, I would be going to a hotel and not the home with a backyard. As a true friend he is, he adjusted and we enjoyed the time together. When I was discharged, the hotel room had a small stove so the food didn't go to waste. It wasn't anything like a meal cooked in cast iron over an open fire, but it was still good. He helped to chase away the boredom until he had to leave. My wife and children were coming up for the weekend no boredom would be then.

After leaving the hospital, I notice an aching in my joints. While my friend was with me, the aching grew worse. No reason could be found so I was allowed to take some Tylenol for the pain. This was the first time since my diagnosis I had been allowed to take anything for pain. The reason was it would also mask a fever by reducing it. A fever was the red flag of warning for the doctors that something was invading my body. With my immune system weak and now disabled by antirejection medications, any fever was to be taken seriously.

The Tylenol helped some, but the aching in my knees was especially bad. It began to affect my sleeping as I would lay in bed and move my legs trying to get some relief for my knees. I would draw the bathtub full of water as hot as I could stand and let my knees soak in the warmth. The relief was short-lived, but usually, I was able to get to sleep. I found myself up late and then sleeping late. But unless I had an appointment, I wasn't going anywhere or doing anything other than Bible reading and prayer. It wasn't until the next week that the mysterious aching just as mysteriously left.

When it started, I found myself having to return to my walker. I felt weak in my knees and could feel them giving way on me at times. Over the weekend, the aching subsided and my need for the walker left. By early the next week, I was back to walking without the walker.

My appointments were now stretched out to about twice a week. With the difficulty of getting someone to stay with me and of coordinating transportation and house sitters for the children at night, Lauretta began returning home. I was comfortable by myself as I could tell my health was stronger. I could move about the room by myself, and we had sufficient food in the refrigerator I could eat until she returned. It was the end of the school year, and she really needed to be there for the children. She would come the morning of my appointments that were later in the morning now. After the appointment, she would be sure I had enough food to last until she returned. Her last trip would be Friday.

My next appointment would be Friday morning—the regular blood work and visit with the nurse practitioner. Lauretta picked me up at the hotel, and we went to the appointment. It was now just over eighty days since the transplant and a hundred days was the usual time for returning home. The nurse practitioner reviewed my numbers and said all looked good. I didn't need magnesium, so no infusion was needed. The magnesium was the constant problem child. The antirejection medication burned up magnesium in my body so maintaining it often required more than the mega doses taken orally.

As she shared the report, she commented about my doing so well. She then said, "Since you are doing so well, you will not have to come back for a week."

Wow, a whole week before I return, I thought, and then I remembered a Scripture verse, "You have not because you ask not." I softly replied, "Does that mean I get to go home?"

My wife about fell out of the chair. The team pharmacist just looked at me. The nurse practitioner thought a minute and said, "Let me check with the doctor." My wife still dazed that I would even ask was speechless. I just said, "Well, I've been here more than eighty days and physically, I'm doing fine!"

With that, the nurse practitioner left the room. In just a few minutes, she returned. She asked about the closest hospital and a few other matters. Feeling satisfied with my answers, she said, "If you have any fevers or any problems, go to the hospital immediately. You have our number if something comes up that you need our help with. You can go home, and I'll see you next week."

I thanked her greatly as she left the room. My wife, still in disbelief, looked at me. I said, "Quickly, honey. Let's get out of here before they change their minds."

We packed up the few belongings I had accumulated in the hotel. The car was stuffed, but all that mattered to me was that I was going home again. I counted off the miles as we went back through Mt. Pleasant and then north to Georgetown. From Georgetown to Conway and it seemed it had been forever since I had seen the town we traveled through time and again to go to Charleston. And then it was a short ride back to Loris and my homeland that awaited me. Once again, we turned off the road and onto the driveway leading to a log house in the field. The sights were now all blurry as my emotions gave way. I was home again, three months being away, multiple hospital stays, hotel rooms, a caring couple, and two weeks in a lonely and boring hotel room. I was home again, and by God's grace, I'll grow strong right here.

Toward Recovery

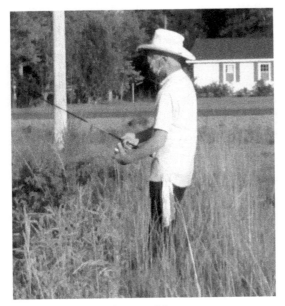

Fishing at Home

I had left home on March 9, 2016, and it wasn't until June 3, 2016, that I returned after the stem cell transplant. When I returned, hope was shining brightly. I was improving almost daily. Just being home had its own therapeutic value. All the long-missed sights, smells, sounds, and furniture of home were refreshing. The children were coming and going, the grandfather clock was chiming. The sight of recently planted fields, the smell of cooking in the kitchen and one after the other, the pleasantries of home settled upon me.

Visits, cards, and phone calls greeted me back home. I found it strange to be back in the familiar. It would take time to return to the flow of the home current. I had to relearn the daily activities of our family life. The children were just out of school, so the new summer routines were just beginning. I set to work resting in my favorite chair, eating some of my favorite foods and being extra grateful for a familiar bed I had missed for many months.

I came home on Friday, and Saturday was busy but enjoyable. It was a day of relearning my home routines and adjusting to being back in my place and not a guest somewhere else. Getting comfortable at home didn't take long. The real struggle was the continued limitations and restrictions my condition placed upon me. There were so many things I wanted to do around the house, but I had to postpone them till a time of better health. With much joy, I returned to my rocking chair on the front porch and looked over the homeland that was for me home. I could enjoy the warmth of June and rock away the time with which I could do little else.

Sunday was a big day. I had been waiting for three months to return to the church I had left. It was joyful to return to the people and familiar worship routine. It was spiritually uplifting to whisper the hymns and songs while following along with the prayers and responsive readings. It took much effort, but the return was many times greater than the cost.

By Monday, the routines were starting to fall back into place. The mornings were the best times to do any simple tasks I was able to do. By lunchtime, and sometimes before, my body was ready for a nap break to refresh itself. Not long after supper, I was ready to return to my routine of going to bed by nine to nine thirty. I would be returning to Hollings Cancer Center in Charleston once per week. That left six days to enjoy home.

Though I was improving, improvements came slowly. My recovery would not be quick nor would it be easy. It was great to be home, but I was still very sick and weak. My medications would make my recovery longer until I was able to get off them. Till I could get off the antirejection medications, I would have to go slow and be careful about what I breathed and touched. But at least, I was in a more comfortable and familiar place to grow stronger. I was also where my mental energy would be the strongest.

In many ways, the next month or two would be just what the doctor ordered, boring. Thankfully, I wasn't in a boring hotel room, but medically things were boring. Every week, my wife and I would make the all too familiar trip to Charleston. Into the parking garage that we could drive through blindfolded. Down the elevator, then the single flight of stairs and across the street to the sidewalk leading to Hollings Cancer Center. We would pass the parking attendants out front and go in the swinging glass doors. The elevator would take us up to the second floor and to the receptionist's desk a short walk straight ahead. The receptionist would ask the routine questions and I would give the routine answers, get the parking ticket stamped to save a few dollars on the parking toll, and then head down the hall to the infusion suite.

The infusion waiting room was not very large. It would seat about twelve people. As some were called and left, others came in. Some patients had a caregiver or friend with them, and a few came solo. Some were bald or wearing a head covering, and others were looking completely normal. Regardless of their appearance, we were all here for the same reason. We had cancer and were getting our blood tested before seeing our doctor. Only those with ports or catheters came to the infusion suite. We were taken back to a room with reclining chairs in which we sat. The nurses already had their orders via the computer system and had a colorful array of vials waiting to be filled. They would clean my catheter, draw the needed vials of blood, clean it again, and then flush it first with a saline solution and then with Heparin. Every four weeks, the cycle period for my experimental drug, I had to give a urine sample. I also had to remember not to take my experimental drug until after my blood test. Once completing the transplant, I had to remember not to take my antirejection medication as its level was being tested each time a blood test was taken.

If you didn't have a port or catheter, you would go to the lab. It was located just past the receptionist's desk. Its waiting area was about ten chairs in the rather wide hallway. The computer told them you had arrived and shortly, someone would open the door and call your name. The lab had about five small areas with three walls and the side to the hall open. The only difference from the infusion suite was that you had to be stuck with a needle. So far, I have never had to be stuck more than once.

Once the catheter was flushed, I was released to go to the doctor's waiting area. I walked back through the waiting room down the hall to the receptionist's desk around the corner and down that hallway to the waiting area. Actually, there were two waiting areas. Immediately around the corner was the first waiting area for a particular group of doctors. Mine was the next one further down. Both waiting areas were much larger than the infusion suite. I never could understand why I had to go to the Women's Pavilion to see my doctor. Nonetheless, that was the place I was to go. I would then wait until my name was called.

Across the hall from each waiting area was a tiny room where the techs got the vitals before being seated in an examination room. First was my weight. Then I sat in the chair while my temperature, blood pressure, heart rate, and oxygen level were taken. Finally it would be the roll call of medications. I was asked about each medication I was taking and how much and how often I was taking it. Once that was finished, I would be taken to an examination room unless all were full. If all were full, I was told to return to the waiting room until one was available.

In the examination room, a nurse would talk with me about how I was doing and any problems experienced. Then the nurse practitioner would come in for the medical evaluation and consultation. Sometimes, the doctor would follow up but usually, it was just a visit with the nurse practitioner.

Once every four weeks, I got a treat—an EKG. Actually, it was three EKGs. Because my experimental drug was thought to cause heart problems, my heart was checked closely. Each fourth week, when my new cycle started, I had to have a series of EKGs. I had to have three that were five minutes apart. In came the study drug coordinator and the box with many wires. Off came the shirt and on went the sticky patches to which the wires were connected. There were only three rules to remember: (1) no crossing of your arms over your chest or stomach, (2) no crossing of your legs, and (3) no talking while taking the EKG, my most difficult rule to keep. Though the procedure was painless, the cleanup wasn't. I often complained to the coordinator who had to take the EKG himself that he carefully looked for the most hairy spots to place the sticky patches. And then he took devilish joy in ripping them off my skin. We both knew better, but that was the only painful part.

However, about every eight weeks, I hit the jackpot—bone marrow biopsy. I didn't find it nearly so bad as others said it would be. The hipbones are flat and filled with marrow so that is the choice place for the biopsy. I was asked to lay face down on the examination table and loosen my belt so my pants would slide down about six inches from the waistline. The procedure was considered a surgical procedure and therefore necessary to be sterile. The question often asked was, "Which side this time?"

I, like so many other cancer patients, had a bone marrow biopsy routinely. Both sides of the hips were choice sites due to the large flat bones and easier access. I usually said that it didn't matter. The nurse practitioner would choose which side and begin the procedure. Seldom did the doctor do the procedure. It began with sterilizing the site. The cold and wet solution would be spread generously over the area. Next, a sticky sheet would be placed over the majority of the hip area. Then the real work started.

"This is going to sting a little." The person doing the biopsy would say. I would fill the needle stick, usually only once, as Lidocaine was injected all around the biopsy area. Then a gentle massaging of the area was done to help the Lidocaine numb the flesh from the skin to the bone. A five-minute break would follow to allow time for the numbing solution to thoroughly numb the area. Then came the knife.

Once numb, the medical staff would make a small incision in the skin. Sometimes, I could tell she was making the incision, but it never created pain. She would usually ask, "Did you feel that?" as a test of the effectiveness of the Lidocaine. Once assured I was numb, a sizable needle was pushed through the incision down through the flesh and all the way to the bone. The bone could not be numbed. So if pain occurred, it would be at this point.

Either a heavy rod or a drill bit would be inserted into the larger needle resting on the bone. If a heavy rod was used, a handle was used on it so the person doing the biopsy could apply pressure and twist the rod to penetrate the bone. If a drill bit was used, I could feel the drill being attached to the bit and hear the motor engage as it turned the drill bit, drilling a hole into my hipbone. Only once or twice did I experience any pain with this puncturing of the bone. Neither time was the pain great, just unpleasant. I chose to bear it rather than be sedated and have to wear off the sedative.

Now that the bone marrow was accessible, the rod or bit would be removed, and a needle attached to a syringe would be inserted into the bone marrow. Sometimes, I could feel the bone marrow being drawn into the needle, and sometimes, I never knew it.

Once the bone marrow was taken, the outer needle was removed, and a tight patch placed over the incision. I would then have to lay on my back for ten minutes after which a nurse would check the site to be sure no excessive bleeding was occurring. I was then told to not get it wet for twenty-four hours and if any bleeding continued to seek medical help in getting it stopped. The discomfort and soreness of the hipbone lasted only several days.

I've lost count of how many biopsies I have experienced. It is a necessity for knowing what is occurring at the marrow level. That is the production place for red blood cells, platelets, and white blood cells. It is the only place to accurately determine if leukemia is active, present but dormant, or not detected. The veins and arteries are only secondary locations. Before I could start on the experimental drug, I had to have a biopsy to determine the exact condition at which I began. Otherwise, I would have a scheduled biopsy around a hundred days and six months after transplant.

It wasn't until now that I learned that the experimental drug was known to extend the QT interval of your heart. I didn't know I had one of those. It is a measurement of the time it takes for your heart valves to open and close. The magic number was five hundred. Anything above that was bad and anything below that was acceptable with the exception of extremes. Now that I was going back on the experimental drug, the QT interval was important. That would mean an EKG each time I had an office visit. It would be read and evaluated so adjustments could be made if over the five hundred mark, that could lead to strokes or other heart malfunctions. I did have to stop taking the experimental drug once because the rate was too high. I soon went back on it though. I needed to take an antifungal medication and one was chosen that would help keep the QT interval lower. The only catch was that it cost about $1,600 a month. Each time I filled a prescription, a special document from the doctor was required for Medicaid to provide it for me. At the time of my writing this, I have missed five days of taking this drug because the pharmacy and doctor and insurance company haven't completed the process. I'll just stay away from mushrooms till the prescription is filled.

Returning home may have been joyful and a huge milestone, but it wasn't without difficulties. I had been away for three months. Now I was home, and a new family dynamic had to be forged. My returning to the role of father was difficult for my children who had been mostly free of my supervision and control. My returning the family to familiar routines was often challenged as new routines had been established in my absence. There was also the frustration of my being a major home focus and now a hindrance to earlier freedoms enjoyed. Though everyone wanted me home, a major family change was occurring, and it was painfully difficult for us all.

The reversal of freedoms is never easy to accept. My two children, being in their early teenage years, only made matters worse. It came natural to question and resist adult oversight. So my presence as a final authority in questioned matters, or changed patterns, led to many high energy conversations. We were having to relearn how to be a family. We were forging our way into a home unit again. Even now, some two months after being back home, the pre-transplant family seems lost on the distant horizon. Too much has changed. Independence was required and enjoyed. Now the craving undermines the togetherness of the family that once moved in harmony.

There seems no going back to what once was. It is now a new family that will be birthed. Everything from eating together to shared activities must now be redefined. Relationships that were understood and established are now in chaos. They will have to redevelop in a new understanding and expectation of one another. It is not only difficult to reestablish these relationships but also deeply emotionally painful to release past comforts and mutual joys in these relationships.

The past two long years of sickness were not just my struggle, it was a family struggle. The family was tested and pressured which brought out some good and gave rise to hurt, anger, and resentment. Sickness, especially a major one, leaves a lasting scar on the relationships of those close to the patient as well as the patient. Sometimes, the scar marks the painful healing. At other times, the scar only hides a wound still infected and festering from the pain and unwanted stresses. One thing is for sure, the past cannot be regained so the future must be explored and redefined. That was a part of leukemia I didn't see coming until late in the sickness. Recovery would need to be for the family as well as for me, the patient.

I began to feel the empty nest syndrome even though my children were still at home. They were growing up physically and mentally. The past two years had forced them to be more independent and they had come to like it. Their independence was, of course, within the safety of the home environment. However, they had learned that they didn't need my wife and me to hold their hand any longer in daily matters. In fact, holding their hand would hinder their much-wanted independence. I was left to decide how I was going to respond.

I could use my patriarchal power to force the old routines back upon the family. I could step back and just let them continue in their independence. I could pressure them to return to what we had shared before, but it would only be superficial and marked by resentment. Needless to say, I spent many hours in prayer.

The reality I came to believe was that they could no longer be made to act certain ways. There were certain non-negotiables, of course, but to make them act in contradiction to what they felt would make me a dictatorial parent and breed in them greater resentment and rebellion. I had to prayerfully seek divine help in determining where I needed to stand firm and where I needed to permit freedom. They had now come to a place developmentally where my authority in their life must come from their love for me or respect as their parent. If neither were felt, I would only be another dominating power figure in life. All I could do was stand on the line that protected them from harm and encourage them to listen to what I said out of love and respect. That would lead to a new standard of my expectations on them as well as my demands they would have to follow.

They were no longer children, but neither were they adults. They were becoming independent. I prayed for wisdom and patience to guide them into becoming independent adults. And I prayed for a divine work within them that I was not able to do no matter how much I loved them or tried to teach them.

Another difficulty of returning home was my helpless condition. I was helpless not just medically, that was improving. The helplessness that is so painful is the inability to work. My immune system wasn't strong enough to protect me from infections. More than wearing a mask, I was continually frustrated by things needing to be done and my only being able to look at them. Minor repairs in the home I didn't have the strength to do.

Mowing and trimming that has to go overgrown and unsightly bothered me. It wasn't major jobs that were difficult to let go, it was the simple things that just a few months ago, I would not have hesitated to do.

I was never the person who wanted others to do for me. I took joy in being able to help others. But now, I was being helped out of the car, someone else held the door for me, I had to be chauffeured from place to place. It was a humbling experience to have others do so many little things that enabled me to be active. It was also inspiring to me to see how far others went to help me in my weakened condition. Daily, I prayed for my strength to increase so I could be the helper and not the helped again.

This became a major education in being at rest. I began to see how much I sought to be in control. I caught myself telling my wife how to drive, which didn't go over too well. Before, I had just sat behind the steering wheel and drove. Now I was the passenger. It took time to rest as she drove and not verbally pressure her to drive like I drove, or at least thought I did. I was learning that being at rest requires relinquishing control.

The grass in the yard was tall so I sought to verbally push my son to mow it. He balked at the pressure, and I fought anger that my will was not being accomplished. If I didn't pressure, he would mow it but not like I wanted or when I wanted. I learned to encourage him for what he did and rest regardless of the height of the grass.

I dare say that the greatest revelation from my leukemia experience was my desire to be in control. Without the strength to do things for myself, I was left to either welcome what others gave me or pressure and demand from them what I wanted. The latter is never beneficial for meaningful relationships. With God's help, I chose to go with meaningful relationships even if that meant undesirable driving habits or shaggy yards. If I was to rest and recuperate, I would need to release my desire to control and be content among the group. I have come to find a peace and contentment in resting within the community rather than driving the group's direction or accomplishment.

My nature is to work hard and lead the way. But leading need not occur in all situations. There is a place to participate by following the lead as well as to lead. There is rest in distinguishing the difference so undue stress and pressure are removed. My painfully slow recovery is a classroom in which I am learning to rest. It is lesson after lesson in how to trust God, rely upon others, and be content even if your desires, expectations, and sometimes demands are not met.

My progress was another area of frustration. I wanted to return to what I was prior to my diagnosis. The six months prior to my transplant were the closest I had come. Now I just want to get back to what I was doing before the transplant. I longed to work outside. I felt the driving push to get back with a hands-on help to the single mother's ministry. I wasn't even able to drive to the pharmacy or to pay a bill. That would shortly return thankfully. Somehow, I had believed my progress would be much quicker than it was turning out to be.

I was told by the medical staff to stretch my efforts but not to strain too hard. My progress would need to be gradual and slow. Strength would eventually return, and my stamina would eventually enable me to be active longer. However, it will come slow and easy. I set out to be active and encourage my return to a normal life as soon as possible. Weekly, I could see little steps of regaining my strength. I found it difficult to be held back physically when mentally I was ready to do so much.

During June, I would go back to Hollings about every week and a half. I was stable and showing signs of growing stronger. I still gave no evidence of the new blood system and my body rejecting each other. The only yellow flag found was a dropping of my platelet count.

My return visits in June were routine checkups. First, the Infusion Suite then the weigh-in and blood pressure check and finally to meet with the nurse practitioner. All was going well, but the platelets still dropped more each visit. The reason could be many things. My recent biopsy showed no sign of the leukemia's return. Blood tests were ordered to check for any viruses I may be fighting, but none were detected.

About the end of June, I was to return for a breathing test and the familiar checkup plus a bone marrow biopsy. First came the breathing test. This was my second time around, so I was fairly confident of what was to take place and had no anxiety of the procedure. It was painless except for the extreme effort it required.

I was taken back to a small room, which had a tiny glass-sided room just large enough for a normal chair. The door was propped open. Inside were a chair and hoses and wires from one wall. I didn't need to sit in the chair and be enclosed in the chamber. I was free to sit at the door and use the hose that was long enough to reach outside the chamber. They were testing two things, my lung capacity and my oxygen saturation. To measure these, I would have to place a mouthpiece on the end of the hose in my mouth. A clip was put on my nose so I would only breathe through the hose. I was coached in taking several normal breaths and then a deep inhale and exhale as quickly and as long as I could. No mercy given here. Even though you thought you were out of air, the computer said you were still expelling air. So the attendant became a nasty old drill sergeant and commanded you to keep breathing out till your chin was on your knees, your face blood red, and your eyes protruding out their sockets. This was done several times until the test results were satisfactory.

The process for both tests was the same. I would blow out till I was dizzy and thought I would fall out of the chair. As I was about to collapse from the lack of oxygen, the nasty drill sergeant would transform into a caring nurse and encourage me regarding my effort. But if the results were not satisfactory, the nurse morphed into a drill sergeant again, and I blew out until my lungs were almost inside out.

My only nervousness was in regard to my past history of lung problems. I knew that at times, I still didn't feel my breathing pattern was normal. I sometimes felt the familiar heaviness in my chest and the difficulty of getting a deep breath. The day of the pulmonary function test, I was glad that the heaviness and restrained feeling was gone. The result was a verification that my lungs were functioning properly and of no medical concern. A shout of, "Praise the Lord!"

Following the PFT (pulmonary function test), I hurried down the long hallway to Hollings. Blood was drawn and numbers checked before seeing the doctor. A quick EKG was taken along with a short conversation with the doctor and then the bone marrow biopsy. This one proved more difficult to extract the marrow, but with a little help, it was taken, and I was ready to return home again.

As June turned into July, a special occasion was in the making. It was my sixtieth birthday. It was most special due to the medical dangers I had overcome. I had survived by God's grace the leukemia suppression and transplant. Now I was home and able to celebrate sixty years of living. My sister from North Carolina and her husband came to spend the day with me. Three of my sisters were able to join me at a favorite seafood restaurant to celebrate together. We enjoyed being together once more and had plenty of joking about my growing older. But everyone was just glad we were having the occasion. It could have been a time of remembering what would have been my birthday. I had come close several times to not being here to celebrate. It was an extra joyful and thankful event as we celebrated my living most of all.

By late June, the decision was made to rid me of the bothersome chest catheter used for drawing blood and pushing IVs. I went to the usual blood draw and visit. Then I went for another eye exam. After the exam, I reported to the Intervention Radiology Department in the Children's Hospital of MUSC. I wasn't sure why I was scheduled for the Children's Hospital, but I was sure it wasn't because of my childish behavior.

I reported in the first week of July and was taken to my waiting area. I was allowed to keep my pants and socks on but had to remove my shirt and wear the gown. An IV was started in my right arm for a sedative normally given. It was an unusually hectic day for the staff. I learned while in the operating room that many were on vacation, and they were shorthanded as well as having fill-ins unfamiliar with the process and routine procedures. As a result, I had to wait longer than normal, but finally, after all the questions, I was rolling back to the operating room.

It was familiar being transferred to the operating bed and the X-ray machine directly overhead. The doctor soon came in and apologized for the delay and assured me it would only take a few minutes. A paper sheet was placed over my chest and head. They moved the sheet back off my face so I wouldn't feel claustrophobic. The cold wet sterilizing solution was spread freely around the catheter site and a stick or two for the Lidocaine quickly followed. The doctor asked if I felt anything, and I replied that I felt nothing but the pulling and pressing. A few more pulls and pushes later and the catheter was out. A firm pressing against my neck allowed my major vein to clot where the catheter entered it under my skin. A patch was placed on my wound, and the doctor headed to a meeting for which she was now late.

As I moved back on the bed from the waiting area, I mentioned to the nurse, "I never felt you give me any sedative."

"I didn't," she said, "if I had, it would just now be taking affect. Now you don't have to stay in the waiting area for a couple of hours. You can leave any time now."

When asked earlier about using a sedative, I had told them that if it wasn't any worse than a bone marrow biopsy, I would be fine without any. So she took me at my word, partly due to the backlog that day and withheld the sedative. I was glad and found the procedure to be painless. After a few instructions and warnings, I was able to leave and make the trip back home.

It was now the first of July, and I had been away from Charleston one month. Physically, I was doing well and making significant steps back to a normal pattern of life. My strength was slowly getting better and a few freedoms had been regained. I was comfortable driving short distances again. I was more comfortable moving about, though my muscular weakness was still very limiting. My breathing was better, but it only took a little effort to leave me winded.

I returned to the doctor about a week later and discovered that my platelet count was continuing to fall. This time, it had only fallen by about three thousand. The search for the problem continued but with the lessening of the amount by which it fell allowed all to breathe a little easier. The good news was that the biopsy showed no sign of leukemia, no mutated cells, and only cells from the new stem cell transplant. Straight As for that test. It was great news assuring us that health-wise, I was doing great.

The next week, my platelets fell again but only by two thousand. No virus was detected from additional blood work, so my medications became the focus. Several medications could contribute to such a condition. Today, we would start with the experimental drug. I had been taking five pills a day. That dosage was now cut to three pills per day. Maybe that would turn the platelet drop around.

My wife and I entered Hollings with hopes of a platelet rebound. The blood was drawn, and we went through the familiar ritual before being given an examination room. The nurse practitioner entered with an assistant in training. We were glad to see her as it had been some time since seeing her last. She was always very pleasant and personal. We talked briefly and then she broke the bad news. Instead of rising, my platelets had dropped by nine thousand. I was now at forty thousand total. They were way below normal but still not at the alarming zone.

She also said that my neutrophils, white blood cells that make up the immune system, had dropped noticeably as well. My hemoglobin, red blood cells that carry oxygen from the lungs and carbon dioxide out of the body, was down as well. And still no particular cause could be identified. However, that would explain the greater tiredness I had been experiencing and blaming on the heat. It wasn't the heat. It was the lack of oxygen being transported to the muscles of my body.

She stepped out to confer with the head doctor and in a few minutes returned with her assistant, the main doctor, and the team pharmacist. I took a deep breath and waited for the announcement. They talked with me about the drop and affirmed that the cause seemed to be medicine related. The dosage for the experimental drug had been lowered for just a week, and it would take longer to see any affect. Since now, the neutrophils and hemoglobin had dropped as well; two other medications would be reduced. The Tacrolimus, the antirejection drug that suppresses the immune system, would be lowered. I had not evidenced any rejection, so they felt safe reducing it and freeing up my immune system some.

The second dosage lowered was the Xarelto. This is a blood thinner used to help prevent clots since I have a history of atrial fibrillation. It is known to lower the platelet count in some patients. Perhaps, with any one of these or the combination of them, all my counts will begin moving back up next visit.

A final response to the falling numbers would be an IVIG infusion. IVIG stands for intravenous immunoglobulin infusion. It supercharges the immune system, making it much stronger. Its biggest side effects are achy muscles and joints along with fever and all around just feeling bad. Some can take it with little side effects while others have to stop the infusion before all of the IVIG has been infused into the blood system. I was told to plan for an extended visit next week. I would have to take the IVIG in the Infusion Suite, and it would take about four hours. My first thought was, *And we just took out my subclavian IV line.* Oh well, an arm stick didn't hurt much and with an immune system well below normal, I could sure use the boost.

Now that I was more mobile and less physically sick, a mental struggle returned. Once the crisis of leukemia was passed, I noticed the world all around still moving at its rapid rate. My struggle was coming to peace with my being left out of the flow and workings of life. I was sidelined with an injury to use a sports phrase. The game could not stop and wait for me to recover. Life continued to move forward. Where I had been involved, adjustments were made and where my presence was essential, things either shut down or someone else took my place. I was still looked to by the single mother's minis-try I had started, but my absence and inability to participate by long distance couldn't bring everything to a halt. For now, I was looking in on a world busy with its cares. I was realizing that I was neither indispensable nor of any great importance to society.

I didn't see myself as any great leader or person of great significance to society. However, I found it very humbling to be outside the living looking in and unable to get back in with them. I felt the returning of early elementary emotions. My mother wanted me to excel in my schoolwork. I didn't have to be a straight A student. I am pretty sure she didn't think I could actually do that well. But Cs and Ds were just an evidence of too little effort. She and I both knew I could do better. I remember sitting on the couch with my schoolbooks opened. She was trying her best to get me to focus on the lesson I needed to master and not lose control and literally throw up. My strong-willed nature and bullheaded determination was clear even then. She pointed to the lesson in the book, and I kept saying, "But they are all outside playing!" After a frustrating eternity, it felt like to me anyway, she released me to return to the yard and play with the "they."

Refusing to be outdone, she turned me over to my aunt who taught in an elementary school. She drove me over for a few sessions during the summer. It only took a couple sessions for her to tell my mother to pray hard and just hope for the best.

I was now facing a disease that would not let me go so I could play. Physically, I was unable to do the vast majority of what I had done before, and now my main focus was on staying among the living. Once moved across the hall on the cancer floor, I could see Highway 17 and across it the buildings of the Citadel. I sat for hours just watching the cars go by. On the building beside the hospital was an exercise area with tennis courts on the roof. I would watch the people running around the perimeter, exercising on the tennis courts, and sometimes, actually playing tennis. I was once more looking out the window at others living out life and wanting to be among them.

After leaving the hospital the first time, I slowly grew stronger at home. As already shared, getting active on the tractor, wood splitter, mower, and renovation work on the houses for the ministry was most refreshing. I was even able to do some appliance repair work that was my trade as a bi-vocational pastor in Indiana. I was beginning to feel I was back out playing again, though with certain limitations.

Returning for the transplant would mean going back inside for an unknown time period. Again, I was on the sidelines looking at others busy with life searching for an inner peace to help me accept my unwanted place. That peace would come from my faith.

Being able to maintain my ritual of Bible reading and prayer greatly helped me feel the closeness of God's presence in my struggle. As I reviewed the teachings of Christ and the New Testament writers, I was much encouraged to sharpen my focus. My hospital stay, painful recovery, and frustrating sideline perspective was a place of service too. From the hospital personnel to the many people praying for my recovery, I had a work to do. I was not left out of life, I was in a different place in life. If I was outside of the living, I had chosen that place. As a follower of Christ, I was always His servant and steward regardless of my place in life. My challenge was to look for how God wanted me to serve where I was and not assume I had no work to do. It became clear as early as my hospital stay after my diagnosis that I had a work to do. I could be used to influence others, encourage others, and even enlighten others as they struggled with what seemed bad things happening to good people. My perspective had to change.

When the temptation to feel sorry for myself came seeping into my thoughts, I would remind myself that I had been chosen for a mission. Sure, it would be painful and perhaps even lead to my earthly death and transition into eternal life. But the New Testament makes it clear that a health, wealth, and prosperity perspective didn't come from Christ. All but one of the disciples were martyred. The first-century Christians suffered, and many were killed for their faith in Jesus Christ. Now was my time to suffer with honor and dignity as a servant of Christ. Whether a word of encouragement, a listening ear to heavy-laden medical staff or a kind word and joyful spirit to those I met from day to day, I was among the living. I had a busy schedule to keep. I was not on the sideline. I was very much active and in the game. I may not be a visible or outstanding player, but I was definitely part of God's team.

The Unplanned Chapter

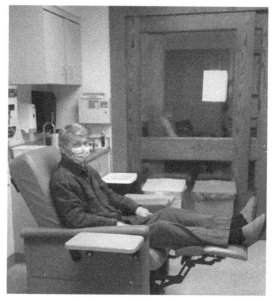

Infusion Suite

I, like my father, am a very private person. He spent much time to himself and seldom revealed any of the things taking place in his heart and mind. My mother was private as well. Sometimes, there are experiences in life that cause introvert tendencies and many times, it is personality. In some of my studies, I was learning about our patterns in life and how many grew out of past experiences. I have discovered that many families with an alcoholic member tend to keep things very private to avoid further embarrassment. Whatever the cause, I chose to be very private and have found it difficult to break free from my private world and allow others to look inside.

I titled this chapter "unplanned" because I had not intended to share these personal matters with the public. It has now been four years since my diagnosis and two from my transplant. I wish I could say my life is getting back to normal, but it isn't. And the truth of the matter is that it won't. If this book had been published earlier, this chapter would not have been in it. Some of what I am about to share are unaccepted by many and perhaps even ridiculed by some. Some are private and embarrassing. And some are just painful to admit. But if I am to share with you my story, I have to let you see into my protected box. If you are to better understand the pain and heartache of cancer patients, then I will have to expose my hidden hurts. I want my writings to help those struggling through cancer to be encouraged and empowered to move forward into a healthy life. Knowing you are not alone is greatly helpful. For those of you who believe in prayer, this chapter will help you lift up, more specifically your family and friends struggling through their own journey. Don't read this and have pity for me or others. Instead, may it move you to discover that life can sometimes be frustrating, dehumanizing, and just embarrassing.

As mentioned earlier, I developed hand tremors after the chemo treatments. It was embarrassing to not be able to eat with dignity, handle things with hand control, and constantly knock things over. At now the four-year mark, I am grateful to say most of my tremors are gone, but not all. I still have difficulty printing anything legibly. I am embarrassed to write a check or give someone a note. I still find it difficult to type this manuscript on my computer. I had problems with the cursor moving around typing in the wrong places. I realized my thumbs were drooping down on the mousepad while I typed and my fingers pushed letters unknowingly. I still have problems with controlling my fork and getting my food from my plate to my mouth. And once it is in my mouth, I have to be careful none tumbles out. I catch myself sometimes dripping slobber before I realize it is seeping out my mouth. It is not a major issue, just a minor embarrassment that causes you to want to eat in private and avoid public eyes. I guess this is the new normal. I don't like it and many times want to run hide because of it. However, it is part of the cross I was given, and I will not let it keep me from the important matters of life. Perhaps, God wants me to be an encouragement to someone else who is struggling to keep their embarrassments hidden, too. This morning, I reached for my toothbrush and flipped it on the floor. Blow it off, rinse it, and carry on.

I am grateful that I can now hold a book steady enough to read its print. My Kindle can lead to problems as I still hit it unintentionally and find a difficult time getting back to where I was. My cell phone is another troubling area. I may call someone by mistake, cut off a conversation prematurely, or get in trouble punching in the letters for a text message. I sit here typing this feeling great emotions and holding back the tears of sorrow. I don't like this me. I joke about it, make light of my mishaps, but inside, I grieve for the lost me I once knew.

As I shared with you my long battle with heart trouble, the struggle continues. The rest of the story is that after my transplant, my heart's pumping volume dropped to about 35 percent. The doctor had it checked a couple of times and no change. He finally said that it is what it is, and we will just need to be happy for what we have, and my faith is helping me do just that.

But in my secret room, there is more sadness. I didn't tell you that during my worst times, I would sometimes get up to get a shower, answer the phone, or just come to the table to eat and hear a strange noise. That noise was my body crashing to the floor. I was not conscious of my falling but still able to hear the noise I made when I hit the floor. The new normal? Well, not as bad but still a burden to bear. My blood pressure is normally about 95/70. Some days, it is lower and in anxious or nervous moments, a little higher. Because my heart is slower in maintaining the blood flow to the brain, I still stand to feel the world moving. I have learned to move slower and stay close to something solid. If you are with me, you may notice that getting out of the car, I stop to stand near the front tire for a moment. That is because I am waiting for my blood pressure to build back up. When I get up to go to another room in the house, I always stop after about three to five steps to stand holding a chair, post, or wall. It usually only takes a few seconds for the feeling of drifting into a far-off mental land returns my ability to move about again. But the insecurity of moving about freely will be the new normal until God gives me my new body for which I now long for more than ever.

Giving up the enjoyable things of life is painful. It is not unique to me. Many know the pain of lost abilities and new limitations. One especially for me is the outdoor life. When I was a child, I hurt my back riding with my father on the tractor. Nothing requiring medical intervention but a continuing trouble. I could do most work, but certain things related to bending over to do something would result in my lower back stiffening and causing enough pain that I chose to stop. After a day of relaxing, it always freed me to continue my normal pace. But with the passing of time, it has worsened. Bending and lifting almost always aggravates it. A day of stiffness and soreness is worth a good day's work.

What impact, if any, my leukemia treatments have had is unknown. However, since starting this journey, it has become progressively worse. I was diagnosed some years back with spinal stenosis. Simply put is the closing of the vertebrae around the nerves going to your legs. Now, just sitting can be uncomfortable and standing leads to a weakening of my legs and a much greater stiffness in my lower back. In between my diagnosis and transplant, it was worsening but tolerable. Since my transplant, lifting much of anything, standing even to preach, or just sitting will leave me stiff and difficult to move. And as I told you, I enjoy our fireplace. But to buy wood would be very expensive and defeat the purpose for using it. So this year, I shared with my wife that next year would be a no fireplace year. It is now a limitation I must come to accept. My heart doctor warned me to not even consider back surgery. It would be too great a strain for my already weakened and fragile heart. So the chainsaw is put away, and the woodshed almost empty. As the apostle Paul once wrote. "I have learned the secret of being content whatever the circumstances" (Phil. 4:12, The Holy Bible, NIV).

Perhaps, in large part due to my heart, a continued fatigue plagues me. As I shared with my long-time camping companion, "I am a river a half mile wide but only half an inch deep." I am able to move about and stay busy but no longer can I carry a load. Work at the computer is about the most I can now do. I have recently been given the opportunity to preach again. Preparing the messages can be done without a physical strain. But standing to preach them often leaves me longing for my recliner and exhausted in need of rest. But I am no quitter, so we press forward, take a rest, and press forward some more.

Memory is another painful side effect. If you remember, I told you that the BMT coordinator said I would think I was getting dementia or losing my mind, but it would come back. Some of it will come back that is. As I was reading over this manuscript one last time, I discovered that much of what I had experienced was lost in my memory. That can be good when the pain and suffering is no longer remembered. However, it is bad when treasured times are lost like pictures blown away. Every so often, my wife will look at me and say, "You don't remember that, do you?" And I don't. When I returned home and regained some strength, I met with the board for the single mother's ministry. We were reviewing some guidelines I thought needed clarification. As I shared some about it, one of the board members said that he thought we had worked on this some time back. I did some research on the computer and discovered that we had dealt with this issue and many others and formulated a document stating how things should be done. I had forgotten the many meetings, discussions, and conclusions we had reached.

I have learned that many others have problems remembering names. Again, I am not special or worse than many others, but my journey has led to experiences that I believe grow out of my medical stress, and there are many others wondering if their memory limitations are normal. I have been embarrassed and frustrated by seeing someone I knew very well. Someone whose name was routine in my conversation, but I would see them and knew I knew them well but had no idea what their name was. I sometimes struggle to call my children by their name. I remember one Sunday morning standing in front of the mirror. My necktie was draped around my neck, and I was just staring at myself. I had worn a necktie for over twenty years and tied it without thinking. But this day, I had no knowledge of how to tie it. I worked at it for about ten minutes before remembering how. I haven't experienced that again since then but sometimes look at myself in the mirror and wonder if all of my memories will return.

There are blank spots in family experiences. The children may be recalling a funny or special moment in our life. I will strain to remember, but it is just gone. At family gatherings, remembering the past is a conversation piece. I am thankful that many things can still be remembered, but many others are missing in my memory bank. It just encourages me to make the most of the moment. We can forget, we may never be in the future, but we can share the present and treasure the moment at hand.

The doctors warned me that the chemo might leave neurological damage. They were right. Following the treatments, I have numbness in both feet. Thank the Lord not complete but just in the middle toes. I have, in the last year, had problems swallowing my medications and certain foods. At first, it was getting a pill caught in my throat and having to cough it up. I began to notice difficulty in swallowing anything firm or chewy. I would have to cut my pills into smaller pieces and be careful to drink fluid with food to make more of a liquid before swallowing. The throat doctor said it was a typical case of the esophagus shrinking and could be fixed with a procedure in which it is stretched. I had the procedure done, and it helped much. But I still noticed a problem in getting my food past my throat. Though swallowing was better, the mechanical part of swallowing still remained awkward.

After about four months, the difficulty returned. I was set up for the procedure again. This time, the doctor stretched it, but I had little improvement. They say there is no connection with my treatments, and I have no reason to believe there is. I find myself again trying to adjust to the new normal and make the most of what is left.

Digestion is another problematic area. I knew that the chemo was most damaging to the digestive system. The doctor explained it this way. The chemo kills the fast-growing cells in your body. Cancer is a fast-growing cell. However, the digestive system and hair are also fast-growing cells. As a result of the chemo, your hair falls out and replaces itself. Your digestive system from intake to output is massively damaged. Over time, the new cells replace the destroyed cells, but lasting damage may continue.

To combat this, anti-nausea meds are given. They can help you eat but not digesting the food and controlling the elimination. Diarrhea is a common problem in many ways. It dehydrates the body and doesn't give the already damaged intestines time to get any nutrients from the food. The greater problem is the loss of bowel control. It took months to get past the involuntary bowel movements. I had to sleep with a protective sheet on the bed and during the day find myself dirtied uncontrollably, a constant embarrassment and dehumanizing experience. But time led to a more controllable bowel function and life without continued accidents.

Another part of the digestive problem involved my change in cuisine. Some ridicule it and pass it off as quackery, but you can decide for yourself. Between my diagnosis and transplant, my cousin asked my permission to talk with me about something. I welcomed her and wanted to know anything that would help me in the monumental battle. She shared with me how many have discovered a healing power from the foods we should eat but don't. She gave me much information and leads on further research and left me to choose my own path.

I began to do a lot of research on my computer and find out what I believed the truth was. I discovered that the idea of being healed with food was both laughed at by the medical field and unacceptable by a culture addicted to meat and sugar. My interest was, of course, any beneficial affect for my leukemia crisis. Also came the awareness that chemo was greatly damaging to the whole body and made you much more susceptible to cancers thereafter. So even if it didn't cure leukemia, perhaps it might help in decreasing my chances for future cancers.

As I was to learn, food was a major medicine prior to the pharmaceutical industry. Many were still using it today, and there was a large quantity of records to substantiate its effect. I did discover several medical doctors and a few notable resources that supported the positive and healing effect of a change of diet.

The theory centers on the immune system. If our food weakens our immune system, then diseases are more able to grow in our bodies. If our food encourages our immune system, then it will naturally heal many of the things we treat with medications. So I evaluated the findings and chose my path.

In all the research, I could not find any evidence that a change of diet would help me fight against leukemia. After all, leukemia is a cancer of the immune system and how can the immune system purge itself? However, it was clear to me that by changing my diet, I could have a major positive effect in fighting and preventing tumorous cancers as well as heart disease and diabetes.

Therefore, I chose to avoid sugar and get off the meat. Raw vegetables were best but cooked was still good. A little sugar or meat, red meat in particular, would not derail the immune system. It was the high level of sugar and meats in our daily diet that was so detrimental to our health. Fish and seafood were usually okay, but the predominantly vegetarian diet was a very effective way to combat many illnesses.

I could not find the information that would give me confidence to avoid chemo for my particular cancer but was confident it would help prevent and combat others. So I began to eat the salads and vegetables, cutting back drastically on sugar and meat. I did some juicing of vegetables until I returned to the hospital for the transplant.

The problem that arose is my damaged system tolerating raw foods. I could usually eat a salad and maybe a small amount of raw vegetables, but the effects of the chemo on my digestive system made it a challenge to stick to a plant-based diet. So, I stayed as close as I could and waited for the damage to heal. That was two years ago.

After two years, I still have digestive difficulties. I am much freer to eat salads, cooked vegetables, and fish. Yet, nausea still comes unwelcomed. It is not severe but disturbing and difficult to manage. Ginger root has become a trusted friend and has helped to enable me to stay on a healthier diet. I stick close to a more vegetable and leafy diet but splurge every so often when in the company of others.

The two greatest problems faced are first, cooking for a family who are not all ready to become leaf eaters. But cooked or raw, the leafy diet is far better than the sugar and meat craving we Americans have come to indulge ourselves. The other is the cost of quality vegetables. Juicing uses much more than you can eat but brings much greater benefits to your body. I hope to return to juicing and will from time to time try to see if my digestive system is ready for it.

So you decide. Research it for yourself. Look at the evidence and determine if you can break a deeply ingrained habit. Many cannot, but for many others who have, they give us a powerful testimony.

There is a walk into my private closet. Things many of my close friends do not know. Allow my journey to be an encouragement to you in yours. Remember, we never walk alone. Isolation is a deception. Look around and see that you are not alone, and many others are and have walked the journey you now trod. Allow others to draw close to you and share your pain. Allow them to give you support. And don't forget to share yourself with others. Life is a journey. Give it your best effort.

Seven Spiritual Lessons

From a sermon series at Tabor City Baptist Church, North Carolina

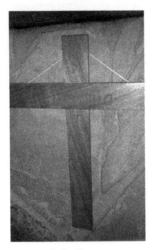

My Cross

Lesson 1: Be Prepared

As you have learned, I am a minister. As my health improved following the diagnosis and then again after the transplant, I have been given opportunities to share my experience. If you are not a person of faith, you may not understand this chapter. I am seeking to share with those interested the lessons I feel God has taught me during my journey with leukemia. I pray that you will read this final chapter and allow me to share some spiritual perspectives with you. I am not a minister in name only. I have taken seriously a commitment to live for Christ as His first disciples did. No, I am not better than anyone else, just a fellow struggler seeking to live the way I feel my Savior and Master wants me to live. Allow me to pass along what I feel God has revealed to me in this journey. I pray that it will help you in your struggles and search for the significant life.

The Boy Scouts of America have a motto that says, "Be prepared." During my youth years, I attended scout meetings and worked on the different levels of achievements. Sadly, I never made it to Eagle Scout. I played too long and when I decided that I wanted to be an Eagle Scout, it was too late to accomplish what was left undone. But the purpose of the achievements is focused on becoming prepared. Prepared for what? Simply put, everything! Read carefully the oath. "On my honor I will do my best to do my duty to God and my country and to obey the Scout Law; to help other people at all times; to keep myself physically strong, mentally awake, and morally straight."

Being prepared for everything is a mental and lifestyle choice. We cannot possess the tools for each encounter in life. But we can have a mental focus and lifestyle that enables us to respond positively to whatever circumstance we meet.

I will not recount the details, but as I lay in the emergency room waiting to be transported to the blood cancer and disease floor, I began to question my level of preparedness. I had little knowledge of just what I was now facing, but what I was being told along with what I knew about cancer was frightening. *How could I be ready for this?* I thought. Let me start by sharing a couple of Scriptures that speak to the issue of being prepared for what we cannot anticipate.

The book of Proverbs is wisdom literature. That means it is a collection of sayings whose focus is developing wisdom in those who heed its teachings. In Proverbs 3:25–26, we find this wise saying, "Have no fear of sudden disaster or of the ruin that overtakes the wicked, for the LORD will be your confidence and will keep your foot from being snared" (NIV). My understanding of this passage is not that God will not let you experience "sudden disaster" or that which "overtakes the wicked." Life will not support that. But instead, we are to allow God to be our "confidence." Our secret weapon for overcoming the unanticipated troubles of life is a confidence that our spiritual Shepherd will be our solid foundation. We can approach our uncertain and fearful times with a confidence that we can get through it, not a confidence in human ability but in divine support. Christians are not excused from heartache or earth-shaking experiences. The secret of being prepared is to have confidence that tragic experiences can be faced and conquered when they do come.

If you are familiar with the New Testament, you probably know the name Paul. He was a devout and strict Jew. He even persecuted the early Christians because he considered them to be teaching lies and diverting Jews from their Jewish roots. In the book of Acts, we are told that Christ appears to Saul, as his name was at that time, and convinces him that he was in fact persecuting the true worshippers of God by way of Jesus Christ. Following his change of beliefs and taking the Greek form of his name, he became the greatest missionary to the non-Jewish people ever known.

The records of his travels are filled with unanticipated and unwanted experiences. He was beaten on several occasions with whips for the "forty lashes minus one" just to be sure he was not whipped with the maximum lashes. He was stoned and left for dead. He was in many different prisons because he preached Jesus as the only way to have eternal life. Read the book of Acts and his letters and look at what he had to face. Yet, how could he not be broken and destroyed by his life-long trials? He tells us in Philippians 4:12–13. This is a letter he wrote to the church at Philippi. It is found in the New Testament of the Bible. "I know what it is to be in need, and I know what it is to have plenty. I have learned the secret of being content in any and every situation, whether well fed or hungry, whether living in plenty or in want. I can do everything through him who gives me strength" (NIV).

Don't miss Paul's point. He is telling us that he has learned to be "content" in any and all circumstances. No panic, no hysteria, no digging in and marshalling our resources, just a reliance on being content. He then tells us the "secret" that enables him to be "content." He has learned that no matter the difficulty, he can find strength in his faith in Christ to get him through it. And don't forget what his many painful experiences included.

So, I lay weakened and fearful of what lay ahead grasping for a secure foundation that would help me get through it. Little did I know that I already had it. I was prepared.

It was getting late when I was taken to a room. After a brief flurry of activity, I was left to settle into my new residence. Never having been in the hospital for anything serious, I was trying to relax, but my mind was now rushing with adrenaline. I asked for my Bible and began searching through the familiar Scriptures for some word to give me courage. My wife grew sleepy and dosed off in her chair, and my sister fell asleep as well. It was me and God all alone. As I leafed through the pages, I found myself drawn to two familiar passages. I felt like a tiny metal ball being drawn to a powerful magnet.

The first passage was a familiar one. It was the account of Jesus with His disciples in the garden of Gethsemane. I felt the presence of Jesus more real than ever before. In my mind, unable to sleep, went a conversation for the rest of the night. Here is some of it, and I will share more of it later.

This time, it was me kneeling in prayer and sweating drops of blood. I was feeling the weight and was crying out for help. "How can I face this? I'm so unprepared," I said. Jesus spoke softly to me and said, "I have prepared you." And with that, I began to see my past unfold before me.

It wasn't until I quit college and returned home that I became serious with my faith. I had started college but was so much in love and not ready to be committed to school work, my dominant personality drove me to return home and look for work. It was in the late winter that I went through an unexpected experience. I was going to church for the evening services because it was required of me if I stayed at home with my parents. The pastor asked for families to go to the altar and pray for God to bless and heal their family units. I had no intention of going, but my fiancée insisted, pushing me into the isle. As I knelt behind my parents, the unexpected happened. I bowed my head and knew all had changed. I would now be the person God wanted to make of me instead of resisting as I had done throughout my youth. I knew that night that I would return to college that fall and this time go with passion and determination.

I had always thought I would study music. I wasn't very trained in music but just had the feeling that music was where I would one day be. I did return and for the first year, music progressed smoothly. I sang in the college choir, took voice lessons, and did well in my music classes. But when I returned the next fall, music theory was incomprehensible. After about six weeks, it was obvious I was not going to pass. The head of the music department called me in and broke the bad news to me. If I could not pass music theory, there was no way I could continue in music. I returned to my dormitory room and wept in disbelief. My young faith was being tested unmercifully. My future was now without direction. I had no idea what to do next. But what I did do was to whisper a prayer. "Lord, I don't know what you want me to do or become, but I commit myself to become whatever you want to lead me to be." It was a few weeks later that I felt a necessity to change my major to Bible and move toward some future work in the church.

As the replay rolled through my mind, I heard Christ's voice beside me in the garden. "See, I prepared you to follow me wherever I choose to lead you." And He had. Through the following years, I completed my college level education with a major in Bible and a minor in Christian Education. The summer of my graduation, I married my wife and prepared to help her through nursing school before continuing my education. But, through a series of unanticipated and divinely orchestrated events, I found myself in seminary the following fall where I graduated with a master's in divinity and master's in religious education. I had felt God leading, and I committed myself to follow. I never thought I could reach that level in education. I never thought I would be a minister either. "You are prepared to follow me," I heard the voice in my mind say.

My mind now turned to another experience. One of the reasons for my persistence in education was that I felt it would be crucial for becoming and making disciples, or followers and learners, of Christ. My passion was not in evangelism. It was instead in leading people to live the way the Bible tells us to live, so education seemed the logical method for teaching people to follow and learn from Christ. Also, my intent was to be a bi-vocational pastor to pastor along with another vocation that would financially support my family. Everybody knows that small churches require their pastors to live on a shoestring budget at best.

When my wife and I moved to Indiana for her to complete her nursing degree, I soon found myself the pastor of a small congregation. The pay was next to nothing and with less than twenty attending, the church budget was small. I soon accepted a job as a home appliance repairman. My natural mechanical abilities enabled me to be comfortable in such a job. So I got my wish and set out to fulfill my plans.

After a year or more, it was evident that being a bi-vocational pastor was going to leave me struggling financially and time wise. If I took a small church full time, it meant a small salary and being financially poor. Neither was a desirable option. I began to think of ways I could make money perhaps by some second and less time-demanding business. For months, I thought, contemplated, and sketched ideas that might be financial gold mines.

As it usually takes place, God slowly turns your focus so you can get a truer view of what is taking place. I soon realized that I was trusting me to get what was financially needed or wanted more correctly. The battle line was clear. I could let God lead me and trust Him to provide what was needed or seek to do what I felt He wanted me to do while securing a higher comfort level in my own strength. Checkmate! To be obedient to Christ, I really had only one choice.

My wife finished her nursing degree and made more money at the start than I did after almost thirty years as a pastor. But God did provide in many humbling ways. Never did we go hungry, homeless, or without transportation. And there was always the joy of knowing that I was where God wanted me to be and trusting Him rather than myself.

"See," the voice said once more, "I prepared you to trust in me and rest in my generous care."

I could feel my body relaxing in my bed. Already, the peace of contentment was enabling me to release the fears and disturbing anxieties.

Did I tell you that I am a slow learner? Not stupid, mind you, but determined and slow to relinquish my way for someone else's, even God's. My thinking was for God to point me in the chosen direction and then watch me get it done. I had confidence in myself and determination to persevere through the difficulties.

When in Indiana, I had thrown myself into my secular work and passionately set out to rebuild a dying church. Early mornings, late nights, Saturday and Sunday, I labored passionately. The result was success in business and church but inner crumbling. I woke up one day to realize that I had worked so hard at pleasing self in my own efforts that I had wandered from what was most important— my fellowship with God. My marriage was about to collapse. The church was becoming a weight rather than a joy. My appliance repair job had become a boring routine day after day. I had burned out and desperately needed to rebuild my spiritual life. I was only opening the Bible to prepare for a sermon. I was going through the motions each Sunday and Wednesday but had lost the joy and meaning of what I was doing. "Forgive me, Lord," I cried. "Lord, show me the way back to you."

Shortly afterwards, I received a call from a church about twenty miles from my home in South Carolina. I was too burned out to seriously pray but knew that I had to go somewhere and begin rebuilding my spiritual life. It would free me from being bi-vocational and enable me to relax and work on my own personal needs.

My wife and I returned to South Carolina and moved into the church parsonage. I began the new routines and asked God to help me regain a passion for following Him. It wasn't long before a fellow pastor with passion and boldness befriended me. I saw in him what was missing in my life. I then asked him to help me return to the pathway I had lost. For the next two years, we prayed, talked, and shared life together as I rediscovered a passion and devotion to Christ.

After three years of pastoring that church, I was called to another church. It was there that I was able to use my giftedness with passion and reward. It was a time of seeing God do what I previously would have just tried to do myself. As the memories paraded through my mind, the gentle voice returned, "See, I have prepared you to trust in me and see me work through you."

It was now early morning but still dark. I was the only one awake, but sleep was still a long way off. It wasn't that I wanted to sleep. I was experiencing something so spiritually electrifying that I had no interest in sleeping. I was experiencing the closest thing I could imagine to the prophetic vision of the Old Testament prophets. And yet, there was much more, but that will come later.

Contentment had won out. Confidence had returned. I was now relaxed and unafraid of what lay ahead. I was sure that He, to whom I had given my life, would not abandon or forsake me. Wherever this journey led, I knew I was prepared. Like the apostle Paul, I would learn to be content and confident in God's care of me.

Lesson 2: Carry Your Cross

Is suffering an enemy to you? I ask that seriously. My cultural view was that anything hindering me from reaching my ambitions or any illness or injury restricting me was an enemy assault against me. Some spiritualize it and blame it all on Satan. Some humanize it and seek our human arsenal of pills, shots, and any help available to relieve or even remove it. Others surrender to the passive mentality and live as victims in emotional and physical defeat. And yet, there are other ways we respond to suffering. However, the reality is we will all suffer to some degree, and we will respond in some way.

I had been very healthy until now. I did have polio as a child, but it was very mild and only limited my athletic ability. I had the usual sicknesses as a child but no serious injuries or long-term illnesses. All in all, life had been good to me. As a pastor, I had walked with many through all types of suffering. I had listened to them and observed differing ways of dealing with debilitating and life-changing illness and injury. Some became bitter and angry. Some chose to live as a perpetual victim seeking other's sympathy and handouts. Yet, a few seemed to accept the reality of their condition but achieved a spiritually based victory, allowing them to live in brokenness and struggle but with a gentle and positive disposition. I never gave much time to studying why. I just knew that the Bible called us to accept God as sovereign over life and look for the good in all circumstances.

So here I was with an illness that would leave me with a greater chance of dying than living. The reality was undeniable. Only about half of those diagnosed with acute myeloid leukemia would live to have a stem cell transplant. The only way known to stop the cancerous assault was the transplant. Of the half that did make it to the transplant, only another half would be alive five years later. So my probability of survival was only about 25 percent. Not much. I was to learn shortly after being released from the hospital that I had the FLT3 genetic mutation. As shared earlier, it only made my prognosis worse.

So what good could this be? Could there be any benefit other than my going to heaven? I now had contentment and confidence in God's watching over me, but the absence of suffering and death was not promised me. I couldn't leave the garden. The night was still dark. The weight was still oppressive. I needed more help to be ready for the long journey.

As a child, I grew up in a Baptist church. I sang the old hymns and often found their message moving. One that had become my favorite led me into my final conversation with Christ.

"Take up thy cross and follow Me," I heard my
Master say;
"I gave My life to ransom thee, Surrender
your all today."
Wherever He leads I'll go…Wherever He
leads I'll go…
I'll follow my Christ who loves me so,
Wherever He leads I'll go.

The last verse goes:

My heart, my life, my all I bring To Christ who
loves me so;

He is my Master, Lord, and King, Wherever
He leads I'll go. (Taken from the Baptist Hymnal,
1956, Convention Press Words and music by B.
B. McKinney)

As I tearfully repeated the words to this familiar hymn, I now knew what was taking place. I, like Jesus, had come to the garden to make final preparations for carrying a cross. His was a Roman crucifixion. Mine was leukemia.

I had learned from my Bible study and commitment to be Christ's disciple that carrying a cross was standard equipment. In Luke 9:23, we read, "Then he said to them all: 'If anyone would come after me, he must deny himself and take up his cross daily and follow me'" (NIV). I knew the concept but not the application. Most have only considered this symbolically or figuratively. I was now about to learn it is to be taken literally.

With the compassion that only Christ could show, I felt His arms embrace me and hold me close. He spoke simply, "I give you this cross, and you have been made ready to carry it." With that, I once more had flashbacks from my past.

My Comforter told me that I had already carried many crosses that were given to me. I saw them as limitations and life-changing experiences. God had sent them as instruments that would mold me and benefit others. We might think that to "deny himself" and "follow me" would be sufficient enough. But our disciple's commission is also to "take up his cross daily." We are given a cross to carry. It is an instrument of death. Its purpose is neither for our enjoyment nor personal benefit. It is for a work that requires us to give of ourselves that others may benefit. It is not always unwanted or fearful. It sometimes is desired, but nonetheless, it is an act of self-sacrifice for others. I was about to learn that much of what I sought to resist and free myself from was in reality a divinely given cross.

My wife and I had intended to have a house full of children. However, it became apparent that children were not to be our biological fruit. Testing revealed that there was a missing link and pregnancy was not going to occur. We struggled with the emotions and disappointment. We considered adoption, but financially and relationally, we were not yet ready. So we agreed at the age of thirty to accept what was undeniable and seek peace in our faith. We committed ourselves to be content in our situation and trust God to give us children if and when He chose.

Not having children gave my wife and me much freedom. Her work schedule and my workaholic nature had few restraints. Our financial freedom gave us the opportunity to enjoy many pleasures and luxuries other couples with children could not afford. Our home was much like a library with a quiet and relaxing atmosphere. Our freedoms to travel for family occasions were unhindered by children's needs.

At age forty-five, my wife answered the phone early one morning. It was from someone working in a hospital that knew about us. When she put the phone down, I knew something serious was taking place. "They are calling to see if we are interested in adopting a baby that would be born sometime that day." Tears filled our eyes, and we whispered a short prayer for God to bring about what He intended not what we wanted.

We contacted the counselor who had worked with us a few years earlier and a church member and friend who was a lawyer. Step by step, the process unfolded and that night, we went to the hospital to be with the baby girl who was destined to be our daughter.

Just over a year later, at forty-six, we received another call. This time, it was a baby boy. We contacted the lawyer, and he walked us through the process once more. Two days later, we went to the hospital and brought home our newborn son.

The lawyer never charged us anything. The hospital costs were covered by the biological mother's insurance. Family, church members, and friends showered us with what was needed and God's blessing upon us was undeniable.

"See," the voice in the garden said, "that was a cross given to you for the benefit of two children needing a loving family."

And a cross it was, neither unwanted nor debilitating, but a cross all the same. I now had to break the workaholic pattern. We would no longer have the financial freedoms we had come to enjoy.

There would be many struggles and time restrictions, but they were altered and released freely out of love for two children.

It was a journey into self-sacrifice. We were both committed to be the parents that gave our children all the love and opportunities we could. As they grew, my interests were altered to make way for my children's interests. Yes, it was now clear. My children were a welcomed cross, but a costly and demanding cross.

I saw another cross. It was the church I had pastored for the last twenty years of my life. My wife and I felt God's assurance and confirmation that to serve there was His will. We moved into the parsonage and began to build a relationship with the church family. I had become confident that my mission was to modernize the church organization and worship practices and lead the church into including the surrounding community of people not participating in church.

Most any pastor can tell you that such a mission leads to turbulent times. For the next fifteen years I worked persistently in molding the worship and organization to be more inviting and meaningful to the community around it. And there was much conflict. It was only about three years after coming as pastor that a major "town hall" meeting was held. The purpose was to determine if I would be allowed to stay as pastor and continue the direction I had made clear to all. The meeting lasted three hours and not always in a caring nor compassionate manner. When the vote was finally taken, 80 percent supported my staying and 20 percent my leaving. I chose to stay.

For the next ten years, we saw much continued conflict but also much growth and joyful times. I tried to give consideration to the members who wanted the strongly traditional way of worship and not ignore them. It came to a climax when a new building was proposed. Some wanted a "family life center" and others just an ordinary "fellowship hall." Unlike the "town hall" vote, this one came out even. It became clear that the church was not going to be able to agree; the armies were entrenched and unmoving.

For the next year, I spent each Wednesday in prayer and fasting. I laid before the altar and cried out for God to guide me in leading His church. What was the right thing to do? How was I to proceed as their pastor? At the end of the year, it was plain for me that I needed to abandon the push for a new direction and work on nurturing the church back toward harmony and Christian fellowship.

I rerouted much of my attention from organizational leadership to pastoral care. I brought back some of the familiar past and focused on being a harmonious body as the New Testament taught. It was obvious that the mission I still believed I had been commissioned to fulfill was not going to be accepted by a unified body so moving forward was not possible. To continue moving in that direction would only lead to a split and an ugly church battle. I then accepted what I felt was God's directions for me—to love and nurture the fragmented body and leave the judgment to God.

"See, that was the cross of shepherding." I had come to abandon the leadership passion and replace it with a concern for the members no matter what opinions or positions they held. I had learned to focus on that which was more important than accomplishments or achievements, people, those for whom Christ died! The cross of shepherding taught me to follow my Master, to submit to His directions, and not pursue my own. Life has many changes, but something that must always stay unmovable is our submission to Christ.

And yet, another cross appeared before me—the cross of care giving. During the last four or five years of my pastoring, my mother and father were suffering from dementia. My mother progressed ahead of my father, but it soon became clear that my father was not able to adequately care for my mother. I was the only boy of five children. My father was a strong, domineering, and independent southern farmer. My sisters knew they could not fight my father when he demanded to be in control so they looked to me to help. After much prayer and Scripture reading, I concluded that I would have to return home and become the main caregiver for my mother and father. My sisters took care of my mother even after she was bedridden. I, however, was to see that the house was in functional order and that they were both safe.

I spent the next year building a house on the farm, behind my mother and father. That is an amazing story for another time. Once completed, my family relocated, and I began in earnest to watch over my parents. Each day, I would leave home early and stop at my parent's home to see that they were fine. With breakfast finished and each comfortable, I would leave for my church work. After work, my first stop was with my parents, and I stayed until supper was complete and they were safely in bed.

When my mother died, my father would have no part in leaving the home he had built and that held memories for more than fifty years of marriage and family. I would prepare his breakfast, fix his supper, tuck him in bed as soon as darkness fell, and drive the little dirt driveway to my house to be with my family. And that was the routine until my father's illness progressed to the point he had to come stay with my family.

"See," the voice returned, "it was the cross of compassion." I had learned something that didn't come natural to me. Compassion was mostly superficial in my life. I wanted to build, conquer, and change the world. Being compassionate derailed that agenda. People seem to always distract you from your purpose. And yet, people are what life is all about. I never considered it a cross, but in fact, it was. I had been changed, but I had also been used to nurture two of God's children in need of someone to escort them through their final years of earthly life.

The next cross was fresh on my mind. It was only six months earlier that I had resigned my role as a pastor to start a ministry. It was a bold and scary leap of faith. I would be leaving my financial security, my accustomed way of life, to work toward something that I had no assurances would even work.

Some years before, my wife and I watched a movie titled *God Bless the Child*. It was the story of a young single mother who loved her preschool daughter greatly. The problem was that in caring for her child, she was unable to keep a job due to the need to take care of her child. As a result, she began a slow spiral downward. She finally came to the conclusion that the most loving thing she could do for her daughter was to give her up to Social Services and allow her to be adopted into a family that could provide for her needs.

When the movie was over, I made a prayer to God. "Father, if you will give me the opportunity, I will do all I can to keep a mother from having to give up her child because she cannot make it on her own." And with that, life continued as normal.

After my father died, my oldest sister and I were to be the executors of the will. It had all been prepared by my mother and father. The remaining money and small farm was distributed as Mom and Dad wanted. It was during the settling of the estate that I heard a familiar voice, "Earl, what are you going to do with your part of the estate?" It was only about ten acres of land and an old house that had belonged to my grandparents. I knew what was next. "Remember that promise you made? Were you serious?" Checkmate once more!

With that, everything changed. I began to draft plans for what would become Bethesda for Single Mothers and stood amazed at how God was bringing together just what was needed to make it a reality. From people with the skills needed to finances to accomplish the job. Individual and groups learned of it and volunteered themselves to work toward reaching single mothers with Christian compassion and help. My youngest sister offered the home she received that was our home growing up. And the work of renovating the homes was soon begun.

"See, the cross of ministry. You trusted in me and now you are seeing a miracle." It was a lesson in trusting God to provide when all I had was faith in His love and care. "Earl, will you trust me now?"

The tears began to flow. It was now obvious that leukemia was not bad luck, punishment by an angry God, my time to deal with serious illness or any other negative perception. My journey with leukemia was a cross given me by my loving and compassionate Father.

One more time, I felt led to a passage I could not leave. It was the suffering servant passage in the book of Isaiah. As I read through it once more, my eyes stopped in chapter 53 and verse 11. It was a promise now given to me and made all my questions fade into the distance. "After the suffering of his soul, he will see the light of life and be satisfied; by his knowledge my righteous servant will justify many, and he will bear their iniquities" (NIV). It was the final checkmate. Leukemia was my cross to carry. It would not be about me but those God would touch through my experience. I would endure great suffering and perhaps death. But my self-sacrificial journey would be used mightily by the Giver of the cross to benefit individuals and churches learning of my journey.

As the first rays of sunshine began to dance upon the horizon, I fell back into the arms of Jesus. I felt the assurance that I was chosen, not condemned. I felt the tears of Jesus falling on my cheek. I knew He loved me greatly. I also knew that He loved the world enough to use me to reach some of them, even at the expense of my life. I had no more questions, just a confidence and new resolve to take up my cross and follow Him. The nurse came in and the day began, but more importantly, the journey was now starting to unfold, and I was confident and committed to go wherever it would lead.

A few days later, a dear friend who had taught me how to build furniture with hand tools sat brokenhearted by my side. "I want you to do something for me please," I said. He agreed without reservation. "I want you to make me a small wooden cross to hang outside my door. Write on it 'Leukemia my cross for Christ.'" The following week, he returned with a small wooden cross just as I had requested. During my remaining weeks in the hospital and my time during my transplant, the cross hung just outside my hospital room door. There were no doubts, no second guesses, and no turning back. I was given a cross, and I would carry it even to death if necessary. To this day, a small wooden cross hangs from the mantel over the fireplace in the sitting room. Written upon is: "Leukemia my cross for Christ." Wherever He leads I'll go.

Lesson 3: It's What, Not Why

If we are honest with each other, we will probably admit that our first question when troublesome times come is, "Why? Why me? Why now? Why do I have to go through this?" It seems to be the most natural question we want to ask. But, is it the most important question we need to raise?

Years earlier, I found myself considering what I would do if the doctor told me I had cancer. I, being a pastor, had walked with many through the deterioration and death that cancer brought. I knew I was not exempt from the heartaches and illnesses of life. I had even commented to several, "If the doctor told me I had cancer, I would only wonder why it took so long." There are many other painful and life-changing experiences in life. However, when any of them occurs, our most natural question is, "Why?"

My considerations bought me back to the attributes of God. As I was taught in school and found accurate in my studies of the Bible, God is beyond our ability to comprehend. So the Bible gives us some realities about God we should accept even if we cannot grasp the fullness of what they mean. God is all-knowing! There is nothing that occurs which is a surprise to God. Over and over in the Bible, we see that God already knew what was going to happen prior to its occurrence. We are even taught in the New Testament that God knows the exact number of hairs on our head (Luke 12:6–7). Did you know that God even knows our every thought (Ps. 139:1–2), and every word we say is known and used in God's final judgment over our lives? (Matt. 12:36). I could not accept that any sickness or trouble that came into my life was outside of God's awareness. God is fully aware of all that takes place.

I also knew that God is all-powerful. Genesis tells us the world was created out of nothing by God. We later learn that God made the sun to stand still while the Israelites fought a great battle. We are also told that God made the sundial go backwards to prove to one of the kings His power to act. If Jesus was God among us, then He demonstrates that God has power over demons, sickness, and even death. As I accepted God as the most powerful force in existence, I had also to accept that He had the power to prevent, stop, or remove anything in my life. God was neither surprised by what took place in my life nor unable to stop or change it.

One other attribute taught to us in the Bible is that God is omnipresent, or simply everywhere at the same time. The Bible reveals in numerous places that God cannot be seen as a distanced being. He is present with us in all we do and present everywhere all the time. One of my favorite stories is in Genesis. Jacob has deceived his brother and father into getting the family birthright and his father's blessing. That means he is set to inherit his family's possessions and was given a binding pronouncement of favor upon him over any other children. As you can imagine, that thrilled his older, and the legitimate recipient, brother to death. Jacob's brother vowed to kill him as soon as his father died.

Jacob flees to a distant land from which his grandfather, Abraham, came. Shortly after leaving his home, he spent the night alone in the country. He dreamed that a stairway connecting heaven and earth was right where he was sleeping. He heard God say that He, God, would be with him, Jacob, and watch over him going to Haran, while he was in Haran and bring him safely back to his home. The next morning, Jacob made an offering in honor of God's promise to him and stated that God was there and he, Jacob, didn't realize it. So often, we make the same mistake. But if God knows everything and has the power to prevent or change everything and is present wherever we may be, then I must give serious consideration to the possibility that God has a purpose for the struggles I am facing. Few of us will even consider going there.

My trust in what the Bible teaches was now forcing me to consider that God just may have permitted, or more so caused, my illness for a particular purpose. I had just been in the garden of Gethsemane and felt a moving presence of God. I saw that I had been prepared for this experience. I had also been encouraged with this journey through leukemia being a cross that was given to me by God. So the only question left was, "What is the purpose?"

The real necessity in asking this question was not for specifics. Seldom do we know the purpose of our hardships until we look back on them in hindsight. I did know, through the promise of Isaiah 53:11, that I would one day look back and be "satisfied" as well as see how God was using my sickness for a divine purpose. However, the real importance of asking "what" was to accept my struggles as having a divine purpose. Knowing that there was a purpose gave me courage to wage the battle and the peace of knowing God was in control so I could rest in His care.

Many will find this way of thinking unacceptable. Many will just deny that a holy God would cause or allow bad things to happen in the lives of those we consider to be good people. I simply share with you my experience and ask you to decide not upon emotion or popular consensus but upon truth. My discovery of truth left me with only one answer. My experience with Jesus in the garden left me with a confidence that my conclusions were accurate. Now, I was ready to face the struggle.

I had finally been released from the hospital and was now at home. I was able to do little more than sit, nibble on a little food, and concentrate on breathing. A large black pickup truck drove up my driveway. When the driver stepped out, I recognized my nephew from a distant state. He was by himself on purpose. After sitting and catching up on our lives, he paused for what I knew was a serious question. "Uncle Earl J., I asked my mother this question and she told me I needed to ask you, so here I am. Why would God allow you, a preacher, to get leukemia?"

It was an honest question. He knew my life. He and I had camped on the rivers near my home on different occasions. He was also a believer in Jesus Christ as Forgiver of his sins and the only way to gain eternal life from God. He was asking a question that plagued his faith. It seemed contradictory that God would allow one of His children, more specifically a chosen servant, to have to endure suffering and quite probably what we would consider an untimely death. So the answer to the question why was what he thought my spiritual maturity and experience could reveal.

My answer was direct and gentle. "You are asking the wrong question. The correct question is what. Lord, what are you doing through my suffering?" We then spent the rest of our time together looking at how the Bible gives many examples and much information as to how God has used suffering to achieve a purpose He desired. But first, he needed to understand the assumptions we hold when we ask why.

I began explaining my statement by addressing our spiritual condition. What is often assumed when we question God about our bad health, accidents, and unwanted events in our lives is that we really deserve better treatment. I shared with my nephew that the Bible is clear that we are neither good nor undeserving of divinely initiated suffering. The more true reality is that we deserve far worse treatment than what we get. I may be a minister, but I still fight with my corrupted human nature. We need not look far to see the destructive work our human nature has upon our bodies, relationships, and churches. The Bible makes it clear that God views us as participants in a rebellion against His legitimate authority over us. You can reject it and choose to believe God is not real. But if you claim to believe the Bible is the ultimate book of truth, you are taught this principle as a basic reality.

First, then, is the Bible-based belief that as a result of my sin, I should be treated with far worse suffering than I get. Biblically speaking, it is evidence of my being deceived to think I am being treated unfairly by God. I am grateful that God does not give to me my fair share. We are taught in the Bible that God shows amazing mercy and kindness toward us instead of giving us what we deserve.

Contrast that with the difference in asking what. If I ask "what", I am recognizing that I am only a small part of something bigger than my life. If "why" is me centered, then we can see that "what" opens us to someone greater than myself doing something bigger than my own interests, not exactly a welcomed thought by our society today. Our culture teaches us that life is all about me. I deserve the right to get all I want. I deserve the freedom to live the way I choose. I should not have to be limited by what others believe. I should get things the way I want them, customized and personalized we call it. To be in community means we are part of something of greater value than self and that we relinquish our wants to participate in what is better for all and not just one.

Asking "what" also guides us into two other important realities. We are only part of a whole and should not think the whole is centered around self. We may say that we are independent and live isolated in our homes. We all know that the truth is we are all dependent upon one another. Life is about the wholeness of humanity. In communities, which many of us simply take from and do not contribute anything; and in work, we know we are useless without a larger focus. Could it be that our world was designed to be dependent and cooperative? It is not hard to see the dependence individuals have upon one another. Neither is it hard to see the necessity of our cooperating together. Those who disagree still exist because of the benefits coming from those who do cooperate.

My study of the Bible tells me that the world is the creative substance of a sovereign God. He is in control, and He is not under the control of any other being. "Why" questions the authority of God to allow or place unwanted things in my life. "What" acknowledges that there is a Controller behind the elements of my life. It is my duty to live in harmony with the sovereign ruling over me. By asking "what", we move into submission to Him who has control over everything. Who are we to argue or scream "unfair" to One supremely above us?

Let me now conclude this lesson with four biblical examples when God did something undesired, and even seemingly unfair, to individuals and communities. The Bible story also tells us the benefit that was received due to these hardships. You will have to decide if God intended it or just stood by and let it happen. And you must decide if the undesired events in my life have some divine purpose. You know my decision.

One of the familiar stories from the New Testament is about the apostle Paul. He was an amazing servant of God even by today's standard. But in his second letter to the church at Corinth, he shares this insight.

> To keep me from becoming conceited because of these surpassingly great revelations, there was given me a thorn in my flesh, a messenger of Satan, to torment me. Three times I pleaded with the Lord to take it away from me. But he said to me, "My grace is sufficient for you, for my power is made perfect in weakness." Therefore I will boast all the more gladly about my weaknesses, so that Christ's power may rest on me. That is why, for Christ's sake, I delight in weaknesses, in insults, in hardships, in persecutions, in difficulties. For when I am weak, then I am strong. (2 Cor. 12:7–10, NIV)

Don't overlook the phrase, "To keep me from…" Paul is sharing with us that there is a purpose, initiated by God, for what he is about to describe to us. He had experienced so much that would naturally lead to pride and a feeling of superiority if left unchecked. So to prevent pride and a "better than" mind-set, God gave him an unwanted and undesired gift. He called it "a thorn in my flesh." You may have heard others use that expression for some illness or disability they were struggling to face. Here is where it originates.

To our disappointment, the actual weakness is not identified. We know that Paul had a severe eye problem. But we are not told of this thorn's identity. It really is not important. What is important is that this "thorn" was perceived by Paul as a "messenger of Satan." That means that Paul saw this weakness as most unwanted and an act bearing the marks of Satan's work. But before you blame it on Satan and overlook God's attributes, remember he said, "There was given me…" Not that Satan snuck in and did this, or while God wasn't looking the devil afflicted me but "was given me." Paul obviously sees this as an act of the all-powerful God upon his life.

Notice how Paul sought to have it removed from his life. He states above that he pleaded with the all-powerful God to take the unwanted condition away. In fact, he tried three different times to get God to free him from the illness. But what was God's response? "My grace is sufficient…" In plain English, "I gave it to you, and I will not remove it. I have a purpose for it and I will enable you to bear it." Many Christians refuse to accept that in their lives today.

So what was the purpose behind Paul's "thorn in the flesh?" "To keep me from becoming conceited…" It wasn't punishment, divine anger, nor any of the many other reasons we blame God for our troubles today. It was God's tool for keeping Paul humble and useful in His service. What was the lesson Paul gained from this tormenting experience? "Will boast all the more gladly about my weaknesses…" Two little letters make a world of difference here. It is the letters "es." Paul was not boasting about this one painful experience. The letters "es" indicated that Paul had learned to embrace all of his undesirable experiences and see them as instruments of God's work so God would be recognized rather than Paul. Now, I could better embrace the cross of leukemia and trust God to be working out His purpose in and through me.

If we can see, then we cannot imagine having to live without our eyesight. Would we not accept it as a divine curse or mistake? There is a story in John's Gospel that tells of a blind man and an enlightening interaction between Jesus and His disciples. Here is just a part of it.

> As he went along, he saw a man blind from birth. His disciples asked him, "Rabbi, who sinned, this man or his parents, that he was born blind?" "Neither this man nor his parents sinned," said Jesus, "but this happened so that the work of God might be displayed in his life. (John 9:1–3, NIV)

What are the facts? This man was born blind. Never had he seen any of the sights we take for granted. At this point, we can safely assume he is over twenty years old. Jesus's disciples were voicing the common ideas of their society. If something bad and unwanted occurred, it must be God's punishment. The question was who? Was it the fault of the man himself or his parents? In a bold and unexpected statement, Jesus changes their focus.

"But this happened so that..." Jesus was directing His disciples' attention to something they had not even considered. God just might have a purpose for this man's blindness. What a revolutionary thought. Jesus says that this man's twenty plus years of torment, to use Paul's word, was for a specific purpose. And what is that purpose?

"That the work of God might be displayed in his life." All these years of suffering by this man's parents and this man himself was for a purpose God intended to fulfill that very day. Its focus was to put the spotlight upon Jesus and reveal a loving and powerful God in contrast to a ruthless and judgmental God.

Jesus then heals the man of his blindness. That leads to a major stir in the community. The story concludes with the man being introduced to the One who had healed him and his pronouncement of faith in Jesus being God's Son. Could it be that many of the unwanted things in our lives are things God wants us to use to give Him glory?

The next example is even harder to accept. Jesus had a special closeness to Lazarus and his two sisters. They lived just a few miles from Jerusalem, and Jesus spent time on several occasions with them. Lazarus falls sick and his sisters send word to Jesus in hopes that Jesus will come and make Lazarus well. Jesus, being several days travel time away, doesn't hurry but actually stays where He is for a few more days.

Finally, Jesus goes to Bethany and sees the crowd of mourners with Martha and Mary several days after Lazarus has died. Read carefully the account.

> Now a man named Lazarus was sick. He was from Bethany, the village of Mary and her sister Martha. This Mary, whose brother Lazarus now lay sick, was the same one who poured perfume on the Lord and wiped his feet with her hair. So the sisters sent word to Jesus, "Lord, the one you love is sick." When he heard this, Jesus said, "This sickness will not end in death. No, it is for God's glory so that God's Son may be glorified through it." (John 11:1–4, NIV)

So Jesus deliberately waited for Lazarus to die before He came. Why would Jesus just stand by while His dear friend dies? Because there is a greater purpose to be accomplished. What was this purpose that only Jesus knew? "It is for God's glory so that God's Son may be glorified through it." Would God really let someone die so He is given glory through the experience? He did.

Jesus said that the event would not end in Lazarus's death and it didn't. Now, it is four days since Lazarus has died. Jesus and His disciples came to Bethany. Martha and Mary greeted Him and complained that if Jesus had arrived earlier, He could have healed their brother. They did not yet see Jesus as having greater power than just healing someone's sickness.

Jesus asked Martha and Mary to take Him to the tomb in which Lazarus's body was laid. He then asked for the stone over the entrance to be removed. Everyone held their breath thinking Jesus was about to make a fool of Himself. But much to their surprise, Jesus called for Lazarus to come out of the tomb, and he did.

The mourning was turned into celebration. But in the midst of the celebration was a disturbing question, "Can this man really raise the dead?" The other Gospels give several accounts where Jesus raised someone who was lifeless. Here, Jesus had told His disciples that the Father and the Son would be glorified by what was taking place. Was it just in the celebration of an unbelievable demonstration of Jesus's power?

No! Read verse 45. "Therefore many of the Jews who had come to visit Mary, and had seen what Jesus did, put their faith in him" (NIV). What God had intended by Lazarus's death and resurrection was that many would come to believe that Jesus really was God's Son living among them.

I will only share one more. This one involves the newly formed church following Jesus's death, resurrection, and ascension into heaven. We find the account in Acts 8.

> And Saul was there, giving approval to his death. On that day, a great persecution broke out against the church at Jerusalem, and all except the apostles were scattered throughout Judea and Samaria. Godly men buried Stephen and mourned deeply for him. But Saul began to destroy the church. Going from house to house, he dragged off men and women and put them in prison. (NIV)

As shared earlier, Saul was the birth name for the apostle Paul. He was so devoted as a Jew that he set out to purge the Jewish community of this nonsense of teaching people that Jesus was God's Son and our hope of eternal life. So getting the approval of the Jewish leaders, he set out to imprison all the followers of Christ he could find.

From town to town, families were torn apart and individuals were thrown into prison with little hope of getting out and in conditions too hard to imagine today. One of the church leaders, Stephen, was martyred in public and unlike Lazarus wasn't brought back to life. So what would be God's purpose in letting, or causing, His true followers to face such harsh and seemingly unfair treatment?

Look over a little further in the Book of Acts. In chapter 11, we find a work that goes right back to the persecution in the area around Jerusalem.

> Now those who had been scattered by the persecution in connection with Stephen traveled as far as Phoenicia, Cyprus, and Antioch, telling the message only to Jews. Some of them, however, men from Cyprus and Cyrene, went to Antioch and began to speak to Greeks also, telling them the good news about the Lord Jesus. The Lord's hand was with them, and a great number of people believed and turned to the Lord. (NIV)

The persecution mentioned here is the same as identified in chapter 8. However, note that the result of the persecution was the scattering of the early church. Jerusalem was the center of Jewish worship. Jesus was a Jew and most all the early church membership was Jewish. Also, the early Christians were comfortable and content to stay in their familiar neighborhoods and worship and witness to their fellow Jews. That all changes abruptly.

Saul began a massive persecution of the church and what happened? "Those who had been scattered…traveled as far as Phoenicia, Cyprus, and Antioch…" This was a most significant event in the life of the early church. Here we see that "a great number of people believed and turned to the Lord." In case you don't know, the city of Antioch, as well as the other regions mentioned, were far outside of the Jewish community. We learn later that in Antioch, there was a mixture of Jewish and non-Jewish believers. In order to get the early church to do what Jesus had left them instructions to do, God had to literally "turn up the heat" in Judea. Only then did the Christians share the good news with those beyond the borders of Judea.

There is more to this story. Saul soon becomes a believer in Jesus. He travels back to his home in Tarsus for several years of his transition. In Antioch, the church grows amazingly. The church leaders send a representative to be sure that their belief is genuine. One of the representatives, Barnabas, stays in Antioch to teach the young Christians. He then goes to Tarsus to bring Paul to Antioch to help in teaching the Gentile believers. A few years later, the church feels impressed by the Holy Spirit to set aside Barnabas and Paul to go as missionaries to the Roman world. What purpose might God have in the church's suffering? Antioch shows us firsthand. Many other stories today echo this same purpose.

As I seek to pass along to you the lessons I feel God has shared with me, I pray you will allow God to redirect your focus. Bad things don't happen to good people because none of us is good. Life is much more than a long series of mishaps, misfortunes, and undeserved experiences. I believe that there is a God. His work is far broader than my pleasure and comfort. When I began to see myself as a small dot in God's amazing picture, I began to accept that the Creator is still working in our world today. It is only then that I can relinquish my control to God's control and welcome my thorn, undesired experiences, or whatever else I choose to call them. I bear testimony that going through leukemia was and still is the most exciting journey I have taken in life. Painful and crushing, sure! But to know and see how God makes me His instrument and displays His power through me with all honesty leaves me ready to take the journey again. But there is an even greater joy and that is the promise of the world God has in store for all who place their trust in Jesus Christ. Blessings upon your journey!

Lesson 4: God Still Does Miracles!

We have many ways today to rationalize an unbelief in miracles. After all, if miracles do happen, then there must be a force that causes them. So in a society that wants to be free from any accountability to some greater power, we dismiss many events and happenings as confusing but still normal.

As you have seen by now, I have no problem believing in a divine Being who has authority and control over all the universe. I have based my life on the belief that God does exist and that Jesus of Nazareth is God revealed to us in flesh. I also have no difficulty in accepting that many of the things we are puzzled by just might be a work of God's hand. You can call them coincidences, happenstances, flukes of nature, yet unknown mysteries, or in the conclusions of nonbelieving medical personnel "spontaneous remissions."

The truth is that some of us accept in faith that God is and that He continues to do unexplainable things among us. Some of us still pray expecting God to respond with a nonearthly power that will change situations around us. Does He? The unbeliever will refuse to accept it, but the believer will grow more bold in believing God really is active in our earthly world. So you decide. I share what I believe to be miracles in my journey as evidences of the reality of my belief in the God of the Bible and His continued unexplainable works upon us.

In the Bible, we have four Gospels or accounts of Jesus's life from birth to death and resurrection. These Gospels—Matthew, Mark, Luke, and John—walk us through Jesus's life and ministry. Three are very similar and one is significantly different. John is the odd man out. The reason is that John has a single purpose. Matthew has a clear appeal to the Jewish population. Luke has an obvious intent to leave a historically accurate and credible account. John states his purpose in chapter 20 and verse 31. "But these are written that you may believe that Jesus is the Christ, the Son of God, and that by believing you may have life in his name" (NIV). No appeal to a social group or academic historical work, just to help us believe. As a result, John gives a limited and selective number of miracles and events in Jesus's life. He also gives us a list of Jesus's claims about who He is and His nature as God.

If you tend to be skeptical about spiritual matters, I hope my experience will help encourage you to let down your fears long enough to test the truth. Maybe you have become so protective against and resentful of others' dishonesty that you put God and Christianity in that same group. I, as a pastor, know that there are many who discredit the validity of Christianity. However, I chose early to not "throw out the baby with the bath water." If there is truth to the idea of a ruling God, I want to know before I have to stand before Him and give an account of my life.

I now offer you the facts as I experienced them in my life. Feel free to research them behind me. It is all public knowledge and record. I went into leukemia believing that there is a God and committed to live under His authority. I believed that God does take part in the events of life. I often question why God doesn't act just the way I want or allow us to use biblical formulas to make happen what we want. I accept that God is sovereign, not me and I must accept His control. I hope you can join me in this belief.

After several weeks of sickness and two trips to the doctor's office, everything changed. With the midafternoon phone call from my physician, my wife and I, along with my sister, dropped everything and went straight to the most advanced hospital in my geographical region. It was by the direction and urging of my family doctor. Shortly after arriving there, my doctor's diagnosis was confirmed. I wasn't told then about the severity of my condition. It wasn't until a couple of weeks later that the oncologist shared it with my wife. I don't think the doctor wanted me to know. They may have thought that I would not live long enough for it to matter.

My wife was just outside my hospital room when the doctor, making the normal rounds, saw her and came over to speak with her. "Mrs. Spivey," the doctor said, "I just want to let you know that you can be very thankful you got Mr. Spivey here when you did. When we tested his blood in the emergency room, his white blood count was just under one hundred thousand. Normal is only about ten thousand or less. Once a person's white blood count surpasses one hundred thousand, there is little if anything we can do. If your husband was just a couple of hours later, we would probably not have been able to do anything."

It was the first of several near-death moments I would experience. Only weeks later did my wife reveal to me how close to hopeless I had been. Some might ask why it took so long for me to be diagnosed and sent to the hospital. Some might pass off my arriving just in time to get the medical treatment needed as my good fortune. And yes, there are a few mysterious examples of those whose white blood count rose above one hundred thousand who survived. But those are the exceptions by far. Time and time again, the doctors caring for me have watched those arriving too late, die as they stood helplessly by. They knew the pattern. They had seen the conditions and what their practices and medications could do. They knew that I had barely escaped death by just a few hours. Now you can decide if God was orchestrating a work to honor His name, or if it was all just a coincidence or moment of good fortune for me.

You already know that when I entered the hospital, I was uninsured. I had nothing to help cover the cost of my treatments and hospital stay. My wife is a nurse, and I knew that nurses don't work cheap. I was getting round-the-clock nurse care along with techs, doctors, and many others, and it wouldn't be free. I was encouraged not to be concerned about it. I just needed to concentrate on my health and focus on fighting this battle between life and death.

Eight weeks I lay in my bed taking chemo, biopsies, and an endless list of medications along with the constant care from the hospital personnel. I found myself wondering why they were treating me knowing I was either going to die or be left unable to work and pay my debts anyway. And I felt the weight of just how I was going to live under such a weight of debt if I did survive. What was my family going to have to suffer because of my illness?

Shortly after being there, a caseworker came into my room to begin the process of securing some way of paying for the care I was receiving. She had a couple of possibilities. First was an appeal to governmental programs. She took the information and left to work on it. A week or two later, she returned with the bad news. It would be a recurring nightmare for the next year and a half. "You and your wife have too much money in your retirement accounts, so you do not qualify." From too much money in our bank account, which didn't last long, to too much in our retirement and then too much money available to you due to the fundraising effort, the broken record played. It seemed that debt would be the destruction of what little I had and my wife's future security. My wife and I prayed for God to give us peace and guide us into His will.

About a week before being discharged, the caseworker returned with one last option. It was an in-house program that sometimes helped those unable to pay for their medical expenses. Not a lot of hope just acting "on a wing and a prayer."

I had no idea then but learned a few months later when the bills and expense records arrived that my eight-week hospital visit had accumulated to about $300,000. I'm thankful that I didn't know how much debt I was accumulating.

It was just before I left the hospital that the caseworker returned one last time. She sat down and talked with us a minute and then said, "Mr. Spivey, I want to let you know that you do not owe this hospital one penny. Your entire expenses are all covered." Once more, tears began to fill my eyes. I could go home with not a penny of debt after eight weeks of intensive hospital care.

Miracle or just lucky? It all depends upon your perspective and preconceived beliefs. For me, it was the beginning of several miracles that would bolster my faith in an amazing God that would care for His child so He could be recognized.

They gave me a few weeks at home to regain some strength before continuing the treatment. The two rounds of chemo had reduced my white blood count down to a nonthreatening level. However, the cancerous mutations still existed, and I would return to my prior condition without ongoing treatment. It was decided that a less intensive chemo would be used. It was obvious to the doctors, and my wife as well, that I was too weak and dilapidated physically to withstand another round of what I had been given before in the hospital. So, a well-used and usually effective chemo would be given.

I returned to the Hollings Cancer Institute instead of the hospital where my treatments would be taken. First, there was a week's stay near the institute and a daily evaluation and administration of the chemo. After the first week, I was free to return home for a few weeks before having to return and go through the process again. After a difficult week, I returned home to wait on the effects.

The second month, my wife and I returned for the second treatment. The routine was familiar. First, the drawing of blood for the needed tests, then the Infusion Suite for the treatment and then the doctor's visit. When we reported to the Infusion Suite, a nurse called us out of the waiting room. "Mr. Spivey, you need to see your doctor before we continue." She was not free to give any further information, just direct us to my doctor. With confusion and a heavy weight of suspicion, we went around the corner to the doctor's area. She soon came into the examination room with a less than joyful look on her face.

She broke the bad news that my leukemia was back on the rise, and the previous treatment had little if any effect. Going back into the hospital and taking another round of the "hard core" chemo was an option, but all agreed that I was far too weak to survive such stress on my body. They had no more tricks in their bags. (I use the plural because the cancer unit is comprised of a team of doctors who are constantly in conference with one another, and few decisions are made without the agreement of the staff team.) She took a deep breath and offered one last option.

It just so happened that an experimental drug was being tested that was designed to focus on the FLT3 genetic mutation among the 25 percent of leukemia patients who have it. At present, only twenty-three persons in the United States had been started on the drug. Some showed little improvement and others significant improvement. This was the first step beyond experimentation on mice. It wasn't approved as a medication, only as an experimental drug with possibilities that can be tested on those with no other options and with nothing to lose if negative effects occur. The two negative effects of most concern were heart trouble and vision loss. If I agreed to the clinical trial, I would be closely monitored for any heart damage and constantly checked by an eye specialist for any vision deterioration. She would need our consent for me to become a human test mouse, but in all honesty, she had no other options for us except a certain and quick death. There was little to decide. My wife and I agreed to the clinical trial, and a time was set to begin.

That began a year and a half of experimental drug usage. I will say that the doctors, though very pleased with the result I was having, were growing more anxious month by month. This was only an emergency bandage and not a long-term cure. The doctors also knew that if my FLT3 mutation figured out what was destroying them and mutated further to negate its effect, I was history. They anxiously waited and pressed for news of my being accepted by Medicaid so the stem cell transplant could be done. The transplant was the only known way to eradicate leukemia from a person's body. And it often didn't work.

Throughout the next year and a half, I would learn of some before me and some following me who were given the same experimental drug but soon died. There was only one person on the drug for a longer time than I was. I learned just before having my transplant that she died waiting for a donor to be found.

I have already shared how this drug enabled me to return to almost normal for the last six to eight months before my transplant. Never was there any heart damage seen or any change to my vision. The routine biopsies revealed just a few months after taking it "no" that is "0" leukemia cells found in my bone marrow. Never did the FLT3 mutation adjust to the drug. I remained free of leukemia cells going into my transplant.

What do you think? It is an amazing coincidence for the drug to be available just at the time I was dead without it. It was amazing that no damage to my heart or eyes were seen in a year and a half of taking it. It was unexpected and stunning to the doctors to find no leukemia present in my bone marrow and blood system. It was unbelievable that the FLT3 mutation did not adjust to the drug before the transplant. When others were dying and showing negative effects, I was soaring with new life. Miracle? Happenstance? I think you know my conclusion.

Before I was discharged to return home, the church I had pastored set in motion a plan to raise money to help me through the road ahead. No expectations of raising enough to cover my astronomical medical expenses, just a little help for my daily needs. It became a snowball that grew day by day. Their simple idea soon became the idea of a local group helping raise money for various people in the area going through similar medical nightmares. As other churches learned of the effort, they too wanted to help. Before long, there were churches from different denominations and people from different churches experiencing a unity seldom enjoyed as they planned, worked, and anticipated helping someone they knew and cared about.

The day was set and all preparations were made. I had only been home a few weeks and was still very weak. I wanted to go thank them in person, but better judgment was to not risk my health by getting out in the weather and among any large group of people.

I still hear exciting stories from those who were there. They started early with many cookers heating up. Out came the tables and large stack of sides to go along with the barbecue. The large tent was up and a large crowd was moving about in preparation for serving the meal. Plates were passed down a line of servers and carried to those gathered under the tent. Drinks were served and all contributions were a volunteer gift. That's when the miracle grew.

Someone drove around the church where a place to pick up a plate was located. They handed the server a check with a "I just wanted to help" and drove away without a plate. The check was for $1,000. It was the first of several that day. The food was gone and still people wanted to help by giving. There was a unique spirit of joy and unity by those participating.

Afterward, the gifts were counted and deposited in the church bank account for use as my wife and I felt needed. When I heard the total, I once more had eyes filled with tears. The total was an unbelievable $25,000. Who was I to have such an overflowing generosity poured upon me? That money was what enabled my family to survive for the next year and a half, right up to my transplant.

I believe God has poured out His blessing upon me through a miracle of Christian unity and human generosity. From the workers to the food given to the many contributing toward my great need, I say it was a miracle. Never have I known so many churches, denominations, and individuals working in harmony with each other. Never have I known a fundraising effort to collect anywhere near that amount. And never would I have believed that one fundraiser would provide my living expenses for the next year and a half. I hope you see the miracle too.

As the experimental drug was taken, there was no cost to me. Neither was there any cost for the eye exams and constant EKGs taken. But still, there was the cost of other things associated with my routine trip to the cancer institute. It soon grew to $10,000, $30,000, and kept climbing. The medical bill came monthly, and the amount steadily grew. Every effort we made to get coverage through Medicaid seemed to be lost in confusion and frustration. On top of the frustration was the growing concern over the return of the leukemia and ever-growing medical bills.

I now share with you two things I believe to be miracles. First is the adoption of our two children. We often wondered why we were not able to have biological children and then later why the doors to adoption seem to be closed. When the door did open, my wife and I were forty-five years old. At that age, we should have had children in college or on their own. Instead, we were fifty-eight years old with children just moving into high school. Plan or coincidence?

After over a year of papers, decisions, and further investigations, I was given an appointment with a Medicaid consultant. She reviewed my papers and asked for just one more paper before making the final decision. To my great disappointment and unexpected surprise, the repeat performance was, "You do not qualify." She sent us over to another consultant who asked about our children. "Yes," we said, "they are in the eighth and ninth grade." She then informed us that because we had children in school, we could qualify for Medicaid under another program. I would get medical coverage along with each member of my family. Yes, I began to cry again.

Were it not for our infertility and delayed adoption of our children, I would not have qualified for Medicaid coverage and more than likely would not be sharing this story with you. Divine arrangement? Just amazing timing?

When we received coverage, it was dated back to January of 2015 when I personally made application, not the caseworkers in the hospital or cancer institute. I was elated to finally get coverage and for it to go back to January. However, that still left expenses from September to December for me to cover. When the numbers were finally crunched, I was left with a bill of over $30,000.

After my transplant, when it was apparent that I was showing signs of surviving and an obvious inability to pay such a debt, the caseworker called to propose a solution. She said that there was an "in-house" program that helped those not able to pay their medical bills. Sound familiar? She helped me gather the information needed and send it to the overseeing body. I was to wait several weeks for a response. Finally, the letter came. I opened it cautiously and fearfully.

"Dear, Mr. Spivey," the letter read. "We are pleased to inform you that all of your medical expenses will be covered under our program." Instead of crying this time, I shouted. Eight weeks in the hospital and two chemo treatments. A year and a half of continued treatments. A stem cell transplant and all the complications associated with it, and I owed nothing. It had all been covered. Call it what you wish, but to me, it will always be a miracle from above. Wow!

AML is a disease that requires the replacing of your bone marrow. In some other cases, the transplant can be used from some of your own stem cells. However, as in my case, my stem cells themselves were corrupted so I had to get my new blood system from someone else. The doctors told me that it would probably come from a national, and only if necessary international, donor bank. Even though I had four sisters, the probability of any of them matching was only 25 percent. So, only my siblings would be tested, and they didn't expect anything positive. After all, there are ten markers they looked for and matching perfectly is more than very unlikely.

All my sisters were eager and willing to help me however they could. Their test packets were completed and returned by mail to the testing center. I had gone into the hospital due to changing my heart medications in preparation for the transplant. The doctor came into my room with a smile on his face. "We have received the results from three of your sisters," he said. "Two did not match as we expected, but the third matched perfectly." Emotionally, it was like a wall of water crashing down on me. The transplant would happen, and it would be my own sister who would give me continued life.

The doctor left the room and informed the nurses of our conversation and that they were to give all the privacy they could and not be concerned by the irregularity of my heart. Yes, I did! I cried and gave thanks for a miracle that my own sister would be my gift of life to me. I called her breaking with emotion as I tried to tell her. Now I could begin to refocus on the coming transplant.

It was the next day when the doctor returned. "Mr. Spivey, we received the results from your fourth sister, and she too is a perfect match." Two of four sisters and all with only a 25 percent chance of being close. The doctors chose to go with my older sister due to her not having given birth to children.

I therefore have become the twin of my older sister. And the rest, I have already told you. What slim possibilities. What unexpected results. What a medical long shot. Was it a work of God or just one of our humanly amazing situations?

My darkest hour came during the post-transplant hospital stay. The transplant had gone well. I was staying in a comfortable place in the hospitality of newly made friends who knew little about me and my family. They graciously opened their home and hearts to me and my family, making the difficult journey much less burdensome.

After a few weeks, the nagging temperature spikes each evening grew to where the doctors wanted a closer investigation of the condition. You may recall how all seemed well for the first day or two. But soon, it was as if a knitted sweater began to unravel, faster and faster as it went. Daily trips for X-rays and routine CT scans marked my days. My lungs were being overtaken by inflammation, and nothing was slowing it. My oxygen level kept dropping and up went the compressed oxygen to compensate for it. When I reached the full capacity, the doctors began to lose hope. My kidneys were failing, and nothing was improving them. My heart was evidencing signs of stress and a coming failure. My leukemia doctors who were the head over all my medical treatment raised the flag of surrender. In about twelve hours, all four teams came into my room and gave me the same message. "Mr. Spivey, we have done all we can, and your condition is not improving. We are sorry, but there is nothing more we can do."

My wife was with me, and we felt the dark blanket of death being pulled up over me. My room was now a somber place. The nursing staff entered with a sad and heavy spirit. It was late afternoon, and we silently took in the reality that was undeniable. Death was here. We had fought long and hard, but it was now time to cease the fighting.

I was not afraid to die. My faith gave me the peace to trust. God is my Shepherd and if it is His will that I graduate to a perfect world, I am ready to go. But it would not be without the grieving of what I would miss among my family and friends. Honestly, I was tired of fighting. I was ready to just give up and quit the constant struggling for life on this earth.

I lay in bed struggling to breathe in enough oxygen to survive. Little needed to be said, just a quiet time of affirming our love and the joy of our life together even with the many struggles we have shared. I spent the night preparing myself for what I believed the Bible taught, our judgment before God. I reflected back over my life and saw more self-centered ways than I had wanted to admit. I saw the many personal pleasurable and pleasing investments that were a natural and encouraged part of our society and culture. And one by one, I whispered the same prayer. "Father, forgive me for the wasting of my time and resources upon myself. I wish I could now stand before you with more obedience and devotion." I was experiencing a greater depth of sinfulness, grace, and forgiveness than I had ever known.

As the sun came up the next morning, I was ready to leave. Preparations were complete, and God had given me a peace I had not expected. No fear, no anger over the undone things left behind. I was now focused on the highest hope of the Christian message, being with God, face to face, and seeing the faithful to whom I had said earthly good-byes.

With great emotions and many tears, my wife wrote down my final wishes. She was planning to leave that day and my long-time and closest friend was to come for a few days to relieve her. I told her that little more could be done than to await the guardian angel that would escort me home. I wanted her to be with my two children so they would not be without their mother when they learned of my death. With a heavy spirit and a weight that could be seen in her physical posture, she took all but the essential items and returned home.

My dearest friend had walked with me through many troubles. We had talked and prayed together about how to faithfully serve God in our roles as pastor as well as godly men. We had camped many times and enjoyed God's creation up close and personal. And now, he would be my companion as I awaited my exit. So I lay back and awaited my guardian angel to carry me home.

After a couple of hours, I could tell my breathing was slightly easier. "It is just part of the dying process," I said to myself. Something mysterious and unanticipated was taking place. Instead of getting closer to the gates of eternity, I was feeling farther and farther away from them.

My spiritual brother took the call from my wife when she finally reached home. "Lauretta, I wish you were here. You wouldn't believe it. Hour by hour, he is improving. I can see him getting better with my own eyes." And getting better was the norm for the next several days. Within three or four days, the oxygen was off, and my oxygen level was normal again. I still had all the weakness and side effects from the medical trauma of the last month. But he who was given up for dead was now very much alive. My wife and children returned a few days later, and the atmosphere in my room was tremendously different than when she had left.

Miracle or "spontaneous remission? Admittedly, the medical staff had lost hope. They had admitted that if I improved, it would not be due to any of their efforts. For me, I would until my death be a walking miracle just as much as Lazarus and the widow's son at Nain and the young girl, which Jesus brought back to life.

As a side note, I found that experience to greatly rearrange my perspective of life. When I returned home, many of the pleasures and earthly interests were now insignificant. My every minute and every ounce of energy was focused on a more divine orientation. I had stood at the heavenly judgment bench. I had seen how easily we please ourselves rather than please our Heavenly Father. I realized how often we waste our lives for things that have no eternal signif-icance. God had given me an extension of my earthly years, and I wanted to give Him back my all.

I will have to share with you that I was somewhat disappointed in my recovery. I was so looking forward to experiencing Christmas and Easter in heaven. I was thirsting to get to see Jesus as the early disciples had. I was ready to see my mother and father, grandparents, and the many others I knew would be there. It was a sadness of miss-ing the eternal events. So there are moments when I look around at my life and thank God that I am still here. However, there are also moments when in my quiet time with God I catch myself saying with a note of sadness, "Lord, how much am I missing in heaven?"

There are other things that I could tell you, but I do not want to drag out the point. I am reminded each morning that every day is a miracle gift from God. Every time I am able to help out with Bethesda for Single Mothers, guide others through the Parental Disciplemakers process, or now preach or lead Bible studies, I am experiencing a miracle. I am sometimes told, "You need to slow down. After all, you deserve a restful and relaxing life now." And each time I hear it, I recall standing at the gateway to eternity and how unprepared I had been. I will push and strive to do everything I can because I better realize that life is short, but eternity lasts forever. I can live as I please, but I will have to give an account for all I do. I choose to be better prepared the next time.

Lesson 5: A Tool in the Master's Hand

In the garden of my monuments of faith, I have a metal mon-ument that is made of many pieces melted together by the intense heat of God's work in my life. Through struggles, disappointments, frustrations, and pressure, I came to embrace what is clearly, to me anyway, taught to us in the Bible. The motto etched upon that monu-ment is this, "We are to be a tool God uses to do His kingdom's work."

No, I don't actually have a garden of faith monuments literally. However, I do have a set of beliefs that are my foundation for understanding and responding to life. We all do! Mine, like many other Christians, have come as a result of study and experience. I have found in my study of the Bible two foundational truths that undergird this belief in my life.

First is the teaching and that demonstrated through many biblical characters. It is my life being intended by my Creator as an instrument of His use. I grew up with a desire and determination to get what was of interest to me and please self above all else. That is our human nature. As I began my journey as a believer in Jesus as God's Son, I was soon confronted with my false assumption. There is much said in the Bible about our denying ourselves and sacrificing earthly interests for greater eternal interests. So time and again God, the Master Blacksmith, placed my metal into his hot bed of coals and placed me on the anvil and slowly shaped my understanding with the hammer of His Word. I saw how the Bible is full of those whom God called, molded, and sent out to serve Him rather than live for their own interests.

Glance back at the Old Testament. Adam and Eve were created to be human companions with God. They lost their status because of their self-interests. Abraham, I am sure, would have rather stayed with his family and not become an isolated stranger in some unknown land. But he left in response to a blessing God promised him if he would be obedient, which required abandoning his own interests. What about Joseph? When sold into slavery by his brothers, he didn't respond in anger and bitterness. He instead committed himself to use his God-given abilities for the benefit of those around him. He later told his brothers that it was really God who sent him into Egypt in order to prepare for his family's survival. It is very clear that Moses had no desire to return to Egypt. He also didn't feel he could be used of God to turn a nation of slaves into a powerful people. But giving up of his own agenda and desires made him one of the greatest men in the Bible. King David, as we know, struggled and sometimes lost his battle with self. However, his story shows us how his sacrifice and devotion in being used by God made him Israel's greatest king. On and on, we could go. What about the New Testament?

The ultimate is, of course, Jesus. In John 3:16, Jesus was actually with God the Father prior to coming to earth. Can we even attempt to imagine what He gave up to offer us participation into God's eternal family? But look at the disciples. It was Peter who said to Jesus that he and the others had given up all that they had to follow Him. Yes, there was a selfish motive at first. But following Jesus's resurrection, these men with political motives became instruments of Christ for a kingdom purpose that led to great suffering and sacrifice. The apostle Paul tells us in numerous places of the things he sacrificed in order to fulfill Christ's appointment for him. I sometimes think of Timothy, Paul's spiritual son and companion. He left his family and familiar homeland to travel with Paul and be used in establishing churches all over the Roman Empire. We never hear of his going back to his hometown or being with his family again. There were the women who went with Jesus and his many followers. We are told that they traveled with them and used their own resources to provide food for Jesus and His disciples. What about Luke? He gave up a medical practice to travel with Paul. He is credited with the writing of the Gospel of Luke and the book of Acts. These important contributions to our Bible came through much study, experience, and investigation as Luke tells us.

As you can see, I felt the melting heat, the hard anvil, and the molding blasts of the Master Blacksmith at work. I came to accept what I found to be a basic biblical principle. We are not humans making the most of an earthly experience. We are instead beings created by God for a purpose and intent He has designed for each of our lives. My job is to open myself to God's guiding hand and experience a depth of meaning that far surpasses selfish wants.

With the reality that I was put here with a purpose that is beyond my selfish interests comes the second purpose. At the center of living is the kingdom of God. Why were Adam and Eve created? To be God's people in fellowship with Him. You can trace this truth throughout the Bible.

What was the purpose of God's promise and blessing upon Abraham? It was to be in fellowship with God and establish a nation of people who lived in harmony with God. Why was Moses sent to bring the Jews out of Egypt? It wasn't because they were slaves. It was to bring about the promise made to Abraham and make of them

God's own special people. Why the Ten Commandments? Why the laws of Numbers and Deuteronomy? Why the chastisement by the prophets? Why the restoring of a nation destroyed and exiled to Babylon? There is one answer to them all, God was seeking to create a people who loved Him and lived in fellowship with Him. It seems He never gives up no matter how often humanity fails.

Back to the New Testament. Why did Jesus come to earth, according to John 3:16? Why the years of teaching, miracle working, and modeling by Jesus? Why the suffering, death, and resurrection of Christ? Why were the early disciples sent out in Jesus's name? Why was Paul appointed as "an apostle to the Gentiles?" Why the sacrifice and selfless living of Jesus's followers? Because God wants us who He created to be His special community. Look at the social framework and instructions given to the Jews. Look at the directions given to the early church. Look, look, look and you will find that God is at work gathering to Himself a people who will love and walk with Him through life. I am here to be a divine instrument. My work of life is first to love and fellowship with God. Second, I am to encourage and help further the expansion of a kingdom of people for God. But to do so, I must deny myself and take up my cross daily and follow Christ (See Luke 9:23).

At the conclusion of John's Gospel, we read about a very personal encounter Jesus has with Peter. Peter had denied knowing Jesus three times to keep from being persecuted due to his association with Jesus. After Jesus's resurrection, He comes to his disciples who had been fishing all night. After a campfire breakfast of fish, Jesus steps aside with Peter for a few personal words. If you will take a copy of the Bible, or New Testament and turn to John 21:15 and following, you can read the account. Three times Jesus asks Peter, "Simon, son of John, do you love me?" Each time, Peter responds, "Yes, Lord, you know that I love you." What you may not know is that the words for love in the original language are not all the same. Jesus asks twice with a uniquely Christian version of the word love that indicated a sacrificing of self for the benefit of someone else. Each time, Peter responded with a word that meant a brotherly kind of love. The last time Jesus uses the word Peter used and Peter replied using the same word. Perhaps Peter remembered his many bold statements about his unequaled devotion to Jesus. Perhaps he felt too much of a failure to pledge his selfless love to Jesus. Whichever, Jesus drops to Peter's level of love and starts there to rebuild their relationship.

Another important element to note is the words "feed" and "take care of" in Jesus's response to Peter's declaration of brotherly love. The NIV does well in bringing out the idea behind the original words. First, Jesus calls Peter to feed or more specifically to take the sheep out to pasture or give them their food. This is the word Jesus used the first and third time. The second response by Jesus is a different word. This word focuses on the shepherd's role of watching over and caring for the sheep.

Here is my point. Jesus's marching orders for Peter was to nurture and promote people who belonged to Christ. It would be easy for us to say, "Well, that was for Peter and not us." I don't think you can show that from the Bible though. First is the Great Commission in Matthew 28. Jesus leaves His followers the commission to be followed in His physical absence. They were to teach all people groups how to live accepted and in harmony with God, just as Jesus had taught them. Don't overlook the "everything I have commanded you" clause. Look at what Jesus taught in the Gospel accounts. Look at what Paul, Peter, James, and John teach in their writings, and you will find a clear track that Jesus expects us to invest our lives in worshipping Him and also encouraging His Kingdom's growth. Not all are to be pastors, but all are to help shepherd. Not all sit in places of authority and responsibility but all must encourage and nurture the faith in those around them.

I have spent much time trying to help you see something foundational and pressing to me. I believe that the work to which each Christian is called is the work of being a disciple and encouraging the growth of God's kingdom's people. Only if you understand the importance of this monumental belief in my life will you be able to grasp the stories I share with you.

As that first night in the hospital, after receiving the diagnosis of leukemia, set the course for whatever would follow I now knew I had a purpose. It was to be used of God to promote His kingdom through my journey. Now I could turn my eyes from the suffering and the discomforts to what opportunities were before me due to my situation. I was now free to serve, which became greatly important in rising above my self-pity and suffering.

My first week was filled with the cards, calls, and comments of many. My wife started a site on CaringBridge that would enable us to keep people updated on my condition and give us the joy of reading their responses. It became a highlight almost daily to check the site and read the notes of encouragement and support. As I came through the night of struggle and settled into the treatment phase, I was very aware of the many Christian friends who were struggling with my being sick. I was only fifty-eight years old after all. The ministry to single mothers was just beginning, and it had seemed that God had put His hand of blessing upon me. I felt my brothers and sisters needed to hear from my heart. A week into the treatment, I was unable to type out a letter on the computer, so I dictated a letter to my wife. It was posted on the site and read in churches. It was my pastoral letter of encouragement and enlightenment. I wanted all to know what God had revealed to me and to move from sorrow to anticipated joy of what God was going to do. I will not print the letter here but have instead included it as an appendix.

It, as you will see, gives a brief summary of the experience I had with Christ. It assures my concerned Christian family that God is much at work, and I am facing each day with victory and not despair. I took the motto on the monument seriously. I was now experiencing being a tool in God's hand and seeing myself as an instrument to promote the growth of His kingdom. That belief transformed my attitude and focus throughout the journey.

As I was encouraged to walk the hallway and get all the exercise I could, I saw something disturbing. It was similar to Paul's visit to Athens. While looking at the many statues dedicated to various gods, he noticed one to the unknown god. These multi-god worshipers didn't want to anger any unknown deities, so they dedicated a statue to the unknown gods just in case. For me, it was what I didn't see.

Each year, the church I pastored welcomed a representative from Gideons International. The work of the Gideons is to place

Bibles in hotels, hospitals, and other places allowed to help people have a Bible to read for themselves. We heard their many stories and gave our financial support to their work. I had also seen numerous times in my hospital visits the familiar Gideon Bible on the stand beside the bed or on tables in waiting areas. When I walked the halls, went through the waiting areas, and looked in my bedside stand, not one Bible was found.

As a pastor, I could not become a Gideon. It was for men of a community who were non-clergy. The last thing a good working organization needs is a preacher to tell everyone how to do things. I found great joy in seeing work church officials didn't have to push or pull to keep going.

I found it disturbing for those, many of whom would live only a short while longer, to not have a Bible to use for courage and encouragement in the real life and death hospital ward. I asked one of my nurses to let the head nurse on the floor know that I would like to speak with her. Shortly afterward, she entered my room and introduced herself as the head nurse. I shared with her how my living and dying were built upon what the Bible teaches and if allowed, I would like to place Bibles in the waiting areas and give them out when someone wanted one. She agreed to consult with the higher authorities and let me know their decision. She did return a day or so later with the decision that I was free to place Bibles in the waiting areas and give one to whoever wanted one.

I sent out the word to the church I had pastored and friends and soon, a stack of Bibles were in my room and placed in the waiting areas. I will tell more of my "Gideon" work in the stories of several people to follow. As mentioned, this was a time when God gave me more boldness than I had experienced prior to this time. So most introductory conversations thereafter, even with my doctors, included the question, "Do you have a personal copy of the Bible?" And if not, I would quickly invite them to take one and begin reading the Bible to see just what is in it.

As I would make my routine walks around the circular hallway, I would sometimes meet fellow patients getting their exercise. That would give me an opportunity to strike up a conversation with them.

We would talk about our common experience. We would also talk about family and aspects of each other's life. That naturally gave me the open door to share how I was a pastor for almost thirty years and that I would be glad to talk with them and pray with them during their journey. I was invited by several to stop by their room and pray for them and encourage them with a reading from the Bible. I also had the opportunity to meet family members visiting with them and be a pastoral support for them as well.

There were two in particular that were from my hometown area. As I learned that they were on the same floor, I stopped in to introduce myself. Both became bonded friends in our mutual pilgrimage of leukemia. I would be a pastor to them almost daily and listen to their fears and concerns. I talked with their family members and encouraged them to make their faith a foundation of strength and peace whatever the outcome might be. Sadly, both passed away not long after being treated. It was an all too common and familiar occurrence.

As I talked with the nurses and techs, the question would soon come up, "Where do you attend church?" It gave me a place to start a conversation about their spiritual life, or more often than not, their lack of spiritual living. Many I found did not have a personal copy of the Bible. Yep, they do now. One was the young nurse mentioned earlier. She lost her sister to cancer and lived in fear of being diagnosed with cancer and dying. I had many joyful conversations with her feeding her spiritual hunger and questions. She was given a Bible, and we would talk about the passages she was reading. I found my suffering to be a most exciting time of nurturing the spiritual growth of others.

Another was a young nurse with a tattoo on the inside of one arm. As she did her work, I soon noticed it. To my interest, it was a verse from Proverbs. It was about being a godly woman. Of course, I asked and learned of her story of having it as a reminder of what she wanted to strive to be. She was dating a pilot at the local air base but not very serious yet. Our conversations were about our mutual faith, and I encouraged her to be that godly woman she wanted to be.

One day, as I was shuffling my way around the hallway, I staggered into the waiting area to look out at the world in which I was not able to participate. I noticed some family members sitting with an air of sadness about them. As I spoke, they warmly responded and we talked. Their family member had just been diagnosed with leukemia. They were afraid and filled with many questions. I helped by giving my personal experience from the previous several weeks. I also encouraged them to rest in their faith. They were people of faith, but the shock of cancer was bringing much confusion into their lives. I took time to pray with them and assured them of my availability to be a support during their time there.

There was also a doctoral student or intern. I say student because the leukemia doctors making their daily rounds were always accompanied by a group of four to six other doctors being trained to be a specialized leukemia doctor. Most after completing their training as a medical doctor would need another five or six years of training to become a leukemia doctor. They would come from different medical fields, but all had to master the set areas required.

This doctoral student was doing the biopsies. She was Hispanic, which was of particular interest to me as I had worked with Hispanic migrants years before. We talked of her ethnic background and family. She was curious about learning more of just what was in the Bible but was very hesitant in taking one. We were able to talk on several occasions. I found my routine biopsies a good time to ask questions and talk about spiritual matters. The procedure was not so mentally demanding but did take about thirty minutes. The person doing the biopsy couldn't leave, and I couldn't move. So I began using these times as conversation times with a spiritual focus.

Another of the doctors was a cardiologist now training to become a leukemia doctor. He was young but very compassionate and caring. I soon learned that he was Catholic. Different from most I have met, he was faithful to attend mass as often as possible. Some weekends, he was stuck on the floor for a twenty-four-hour shift. There was always one of the training doctors on the floor during the night as emergencies were frequent. Often, he was to be in on Sunday to help make the rounds and fill in for the higher doctors who were off that day. He would go to the early mass and then to the hospital. We talked much about our faith and his sincere effort to live for Christ though in a different religious environment than I as a Baptist. I was sometimes an encouragement to him, and sometimes, he was a spiritual encouragement to me.

Many were the times to share an encouraging word, pray, or share some truth from the Bible that would give the weak and struggling something upon which to rest. One by one, people were brought into my pathway so God could use me to share His love and comfort to those in fear and confusion.

I felt very strongly that I was to display a faith that was genuine and solid. Many of the hospital staff were more familiar with those who identified themselves as Christian but lost most spiritual sincerity when faced with leukemia and the real presence of death. I felt the importance of demonstrating a real faith in Christ that held solid and true regardless of medical turmoil.

When I played the recorder, my faith was declared with each hymn. When talking with the staff about spiritual matters, they could see my sincerity in trusting in Christ no matter how despairing my condition appeared. As I handed out Bibles, they could see a commitment to be used of Christ and not turn my focus inward because of my struggles. And a few times when interrupting my prayers, while kneeling at my chair, they knew I was serious about being a Christian. It was my aim to live sincerely for Christ and be the light He had placed me there to be. So Bible readings, Christian worship, and inspirational music, and other Christian materials I read as long as I could were a witness to a faith that was real and not just convenient. I will never know just how God did use me. I am most grateful that He chose to do so and enabled me to faithfully represent Him.

Lesson 6: My Grace Is Sufficient

In our moments of honesty, we are forced to admit that we can withstand far more than we want to admit. The secret is our determination and inner strength. As a Christian, we know that there is an inner power that comes from beyond ourselves. Many refer to it as a "higher power." I think that means a power to do what I must do even when self is crying out to do what is harmful to me. I believe God is that "higher power." My life is a testimony of how I have turned to God for strength to endure and face troubled times I feared to enter. I am sure that most of you reading this have experienced the same. We may see it coming or find ourselves thrown into it. We know that we are too weak to survive the stress and weight upon us. Yet, if we stop, the human determination to survive and ask for a power outside of ourselves, we experience a calm strength that enables us to bear the pain and mental stresses placed upon us. That unknown ability to face and move through and beyond our struggles is what I am calling "grace." This source for dealing with and overcoming our fearful and debilitating experiences is a work of God's grace to us.

We have earlier looked at the apostle Paul's "thorn in the flesh." We took note of what God was doing by allowing Paul to have such a continuing disability. Now let's look more closely at God's response to Paul.

As we return to 2 Corinthians 12, we are reminded that Paul tried three times to have God remove this bothersome, aggravating, and constantly humiliating gift. Paul said it was "given to me" for the purpose of keeping him humbled. But that was not his first thought. His first thought seems to have been more along the line of how he could remove this hindrance to his daily ministry. There are some interesting circumstances surrounding this event.

We have learned from the change of pronouns in the book of Acts that Luke, the author, traveled with Paul. Luke, as you might recall, was a physician. Paul refers to him in his letter to Colossae as "Our dear friend Luke, the doctor..." (Col. 4:14, NIV). Paul is here sending greetings from those traveling and serving with him. We later find that Luke stayed with Paul during his imprisonment. In Paul's letter to his spiritual son and most trusted companion, he shares another insight about Luke, "Only Luke is with me" (2 Tim. 4:11, NIV).

Paul wrote this letter from prison in Rome. He tells of how he feels his race is complete and his earthly time is almost gone. He calls Timothy to leave the church he has been leading and to come be by his side in this dark and depressing time. All have forsaken Paul except the physician Luke. I think this is significant when seen in the light of Paul's thorn in the flesh. Notice the insight Paul gives to the church at Galatia. In Galatians 4:15, we find, "I can testify that if you could have done so, you would have torn out your eyes and given them to me" (NIV). Why if not due to some severe and debilitating eye condition? This does not mean it was Paul's thorn in the flesh, but it does make us aware that Paul had a serious and lasting physical condition.

Yes, I believe that Luke traveled with Paul because of his commitment to Jesus Christ as Paul preached. However, I also believe that Luke went alongside Paul to medically assist him. Acts reveals that Luke traveled with Paul not as a continuing companion in Paul's missionary work but for a time here and for a time there. We also see that when Paul was arrested in Jerusalem and began his long prison journey that would take him to Rome to stand trial before the emperor, Luke went with him. The dangerous journey to Rome is given by Luke as a firsthand account. In what may have been Paul's final letter, Luke is identified as Paul's sole companion in the Roman prison. Might it be that the greatly loved and appreciated doctor had become Paul's personal physician? Whatever your conclusion is, it is obvious that Paul endured a long-term and painful condition.

Let us return to 2 Corinthians. Here, Paul tells us that when he sought God's help in removing this unwanted suffering God's response was for him to accept it and trust God's given strength to bear it. That is certainly not the answer we would want either. As unwilling as Paul was to accept it, this was God's response to his prayers. We, however, refuse to accept or believe such as well. We seek pills to remove it, surgeries to relieve us, spiritual friends to pray it away, but whatever the cost, we want it gone. Often, the reason goes back to a basic spiritual deception. Our culture and human-centered thinking see life as our short time to live it to the fullest. So anything that hinders our pleasure and personal fulfillment needs to be removed. However, the Bible teaches us that we are here to live in a relationship with God. That was His purpose with Adam and Eve, and that is His purpose for us. Jesus affirms it and teaches us to live for our eternal time in God's unlimited presence and not to grasp for earthly satisfaction and pleasures. But we refuse to embrace such an idea. "My grace is sufficient…" is just unacceptable. Therefore, we fight against our weakness, illness, and limitations leading us into bitterness and a lifetime of depression, addictions, and unhappiness.

Perhaps, it is time for us to receive God's grace for our daily lives. Many of us believe that God shows us grace in forgiving us of our sins. We believe this is the work Christ accomplished for us through His death and resurrection. God's grace is not limited to just our sins. The Bible is clear that God gives us grace to bear trials and endure great sufferings, too. During my struggles, of which leukemia was the greatest, I have learned that sometimes, we must accept that "My grace is sufficient."

That means that what we fear and do not want must be accepted as our friend. That which restricts us from the freedoms for which we demand must be welcomed. This is a spiritual principle for those living with a desire to participate in God's kingdom of people. If you have not allowed Christ to forgive you and have not accepted Him as Lord of all the universe, then fighting for a better living experience is all you can hope for. But when you believe this life is only a short prelude to an eternal life, then you have more to live for than just today.

I shared with you that I had polio as a young child. It limited my physical abilities and athletic abilities. I was laughed at for being slower and weaker than my scouting friends. I fought it and gave more determination to negate it but couldn't. I grew angry and sought other ways to prove my equality with the athletic achievers.

I have always felt inferior to the academic crowd. My attention span was short and my intellectual abilities less than I wanted. Once more, I let anger and bitterness push me into an "I don't care" attitude and found comfort in those rejecting educational pursuits and settling for a "let's have a good time" instead. So I did and settled for "just getting by."

I had four sisters, two older and two younger. There were only two bedrooms and one bathroom, which made me, literally, "the odd man out." I chose to avoid the family feminine drama and isolate myself in outside activities and individual ambitions. I was pretty much a loner. I had friends, of course, but trusted myself to no group and chose to let no one decide my direction.

I bundled up all this inner pain and made one bold leap for acceptance, significance, and a place to belong. That place is called marriage. I had committed myself to follow Christ. I had completed my college studies. With the passion of a drowning sailor, I sought for a wife to put her healing ointment upon my inner pain. For a short period, the stress and demands upon my new bride were tolerable, but before long, my demands for healing were more than our love could heal. I tried all the ways familiar to us to make her, not really our marriage, fulfill my inner quest.

For several years, I pleaded with God to fix my problem. But no fix was found. No work of God's miraculous touch was felt. So, it was in my despair and at the end of my rope that I cried out like Paul and heard the familiar voice, "My grace is sufficient." As I began the long journey of accepting grace and living under His crushing work, I realized that without God's denial of my quest, I would not be of much use to Him. If I got what I wanted, I would only want something else, something more or something better. It was then that I began the difficult journey of rebuilding my fellowship and submission to Christ.

God's grace doesn't take away the pain of inner longings. As I am about to share with you, it didn't take away my pain and emotional struggles associated with leukemia. But it did accomplish two important things—courage and strength to endure, and a focus to be used by God more than seek selfish interests. Every day, the battle returns. But each day, "My grace is sufficient…" With each victory, there is the inner joy of giving self for that which is greater than me.

With all of that in the background, I entered the hospital. I knew little of what lay ahead but was soon to get glimpses of my future and "grace" to accept it and survive the experience. And don't think that I zipped through all this with an always pleasant and joyful disposition. There were days of depression, frustration, anger, and self-pity. But time and again, I clung to the words, "My grace is sufficient." There will probably be little that is new here. Most is already shared with you in earlier chapters of this book. However, please allow me to review places in my journey that taught me to trust in God's grace. I trust it will encourage your reliance upon God's grace, too. Let me now share some of how it was.

Those of you who have undergone chemo treatments will remember the pain of what I share here. It wasn't physical pain. It was instead emotional and psychological pain. There was a certain amount of physical pain but nothing nearly as intense as the mental and emotional. As I would exercise daily by making several trips around the hallway, I could feel the life within me slowly leaving. Weaker by the day, I began having to force myself to leave my room and shuffle my way down the hallway. Often, my wife would accompany me pushing my pole hanging with chemical concoctions to save my energy or more than likely to help prevent my stumbling and falling. As I continued into the second round of chemo, giving up was a more desired choice than leaving my room. I would often trudge my way into the hallway with whoever was with me pushing a wheelchair behind me in case of my collapse in exhaustion. I would see the nurses and visitors walking effortlessly and think to myself, *Will I ever be free to walk again?*

It was during my second round of chemo that I was moved to a room on the west side of the hospital. From there, I could see the buildings of the Citadel, US 17, and a building next door with an exercise area and tennis courts on top of it. It was often more torture than helpful as I watched tennis players moving quickly on the court and hitting the ball back and forth over the net. It had been a game I had greatly enjoyed through the years as a way to get physical exercise. I would watch the joggers going around the perimeter of the courts and feel the dark cloud of sadness returning. Tears would begin forming in my eyes as I wondered if I would ever be anything but an adult infant.

Often, I would whisper a prayer of hope, "Lord, give me strength to persevere." It was more emotional darkness than physically painful. When I completed the second round of chemo, I was little more than the shell of a person. Inside, I felt destroyed. The me that was inside this body was struggling to just hold on. I wanted to just turn loose and let it be over with, but as my family and friends would read for me passages in the Bible, I would be reminded, "My grace is sufficient." Though my body and inner being were wasting away and crushed by weakness, my spirit refused to let go. And so it was that step-by-step and day-by-day determination that became my mode of endurance.

As the chemo began to take its destructive toll, I would see in the mirror a strong and independent man wasting away. It was hard to look into the mirror and accept what I saw. The fullness of my face was vanishing, muscle mass was disappearing, and I was becoming a ghostly figure who would rather hide away from reflections that only brought more inner pain and sadness. As I have shared with you, returning for the third round of chemo was a difficult emotional journey. I now better understood why the transplant team had a psychiatrist as part of the evaluation process. I began to better understand why only 50–60 percent of those made it through the initial treatment for AML. When you lose the will to live, your body gives in. It is the inner self that must persevere despite the emotional pain and desire to give up. Just how much can we bear? I was discovering it wasn't a physical question but a mental one. As long as you have a determination to survive and a hope for the future, you can endure more than you can imagine. My determination came not from my refusal to die but from a faith that pushed me forward. I was here to be used of God. I could not give up. I was reflecting faith in Christ to all the hospital staff, and my life would enable them to see the power of God in someone's life. So, God's grace was sufficient and through the inner torment, I found a peace and strength from my faith to take the next step, and then the next, and then the next.

It was during my initial treatment that I began to notice problems seeing. I had asked for some books to be brought that would be spiritually encouraging to me. I was able to continue my daily Bible study and prayer times as shared earlier. But this morning, I was having problems focusing on the letters and words. I found it difficult to see the print and began noticing reddish blotches moving about.

When the doctors made their morning rounds, I shared with them what I was experiencing. They, of course, called for the eye doctor, and he came late that afternoon. He took his light, which looked like that of a coal miner, and a magnifying glass and holding my eyelids open began looking into my eyeball. It only took a minute to give his diagnosis. "Your blood has become too thin, and the little capillaries in your eyeballs are allowing blood to seep into your eyes, which is obstructing your vision." He went on to say that it was nothing permanent, but it would take a while to clear up.

My medications were adjusted and a closer watch on the thinness of my blood was kept. It took a long wait for my eyes to clear. No more reading, no watching anything or working on my computer. Now, I was limited to what I could hear. This was a difficult spiritual struggle for me. The routine of my daily time in the Bible was of great importance to me. Reading autobiographies of outstanding men and women of the faith was a source of strength and encouragement. Now, my world of reading was gone, and it would be weeks or months before it would return.

It was here that I found a greater experience in the sufficiency of God's grace. I cried out in prayer for God to help me in losing my ability to run to Him in His Word. As I cried out in prayer, God spoke and gave the peace needed to be at rest once more. "It is all right, my son, I will hold you and keep you close." The anxiety and frustration were now gone. Each day brought a greater awareness of God's holding me close to Him. I still longed for others to read to me, and God provided several that would assist me in private times of worship as I listened to their reading of the Bible.

The long journey of heart failure began during the initial treatment. My heart rate was confirmed running wild, and, of course, the heart doctors were called in. This began a journey that continues to this day. I could not tell when my heart began beating, like a car's motor running at a very high speed while still in neutral. I was already too fatigued to notice any loss of energy, so all continued except for more medications. The doctors shared with me that my condition was not fatal but would lead to strokes as my blood was not circulating properly and therefore allowing clotting that would move and stop the blood's flow. However, in my present condition, it was best to use medications to help prevent clotting and wait till later for any attempts to put my heart back into its regular rhythm.

It was later that the struggle came. As I began to regain my health, it became apparent that my heart condition was limiting my energy level. When able, I was scheduled for a cardioversion to set my heart into its regular rhythm. Renewed energy was felt, and I began enjoying some simple outdoor activities again.

Out of nowhere, I would feel my energy level drop and knew what was happening. As I was making regular visits to the cancer institute, their routine check would pick up the irregular heartbeat. As the problem persisted, further testing was desired. I was given a monitor to wear for a month and received routine calls about my heart rate being too high or when resting, stopping for too long. I was admitted locally once and went through another cardioversion. I was later to have a third while using various medications to try and keep my heart from returning to its racing pattern.

It was during all of this that preparation for the stem cell transplant began. One element was the pumping capacity of my heart. I was given an ultrasound of my heart to determine the percentage. The transplant would not be done unless my heart was at a minimal of 45–50 percent. The first test revealed that I was only at about 40 percent. The doctor felt it would come back up with a little time but probably not to the normal range of 75 percent or better. When it was checked again shortly before the transplant, it had come up just enough for me to have the transplant.

Following the transplant, another test was performed, and the results showed that I had gone down to about 30 percent. The doctor was hopeful it would increase but was concerned that it may not be much. As I was cautioned, it didn't rise much at all. After about six months, it was confirmed that my heart volume was only about 35 percent. And that is where it has remained.

The physical side of the heart condition is continued fatigue. There is also the lightheaded feeling that comes from getting up and moving. I have gotten out of bed and collapsed at my dresser. I have lost consciousness trying to get to the home phone. I still often get up from my chair and take a few steps and have to hold to something and wait for my heart to get more blood up to my brain. And again,

I would pray, "Lord, must I live under such restraints?" His answer was the same as before, "My grace is sufficient."

In all honesty, I have cried out to God, "Lord, I don't want more grace. I want to be normal again." But I would look at a small wooden cross hanging on my fireplace mantel and be reminded that I am on a journey of serving and representing Christ. I am God's tool to be used as He decides and not as I wish. In humility, I have asked for forgiveness and cling to a divine grace that enables me to make the most of what is given and not become bitter and angry at what is no longer part of my daily life.

One of my surprises was the peace God's grace gave to me in my near-death experiences. First was the return to Hollings Cancer Institute. I was literally dangling by a thread. The one chemo available that wouldn't cause my weakened body to collapse wasn't destroying the cancerous white blood cells. As the doctor shared the bad news, I felt a peace from God to trust His plan and rest in His care. I had preached the good news of a heaven provided for all who entrusted themselves to Jesus Christ. Now was my ultimate test. There was no fear of dying or grasping for a lifesaving solution. There was instead a peace to trust God to do what He willed. If it was my time of departure, I was confident that a much better world awaited me for eternity. I had many things I still wanted to experience and see, but I had peace to let it go. My wife and children would face many difficulties in my absence, but I rested in my Lord who I was sure would meet their every need. The experimental drug was not a grasp after continued life but instead a step into the unknown, trusting God to bring about whatever His will for me was.

A year and a half later, when all my doctors offered me their condolences and forgiveness for not having any way to stop my dying, I found peace again. This time, it seemed a sure thing. The medical staff had exhausted all they had. I was struggling to hold on, and now the final straw was falling upon my already crushing load. I felt an unexpected peace come over me that all would be well. Not that I would live, but that He who I had served would take care of that, which I would leave behind. As my wife left to return home and I lay still awaiting the angel of death to come, it was an amazing time of peace and expectation. What I had preached, what I had read in the Bible, and what I had shared with many by their dying bed was now my peace, it is real. God's grace was again sufficient.

As I finally survived the chemo, heart failure, massive amounts of medicines, and other obstacles, a new hope was beginning to dawn. No more treatments, fewer medicines and now the regaining of some of my mobility gave me renewed hope of life. Now was the time to find out what my new normal would be.

I went on disability shortly after entering the hospital the first time. Was this to continue or would I be able to work again? What would my opportunities and limitations be? What lifelong adjustments would I need to make? We were now to find out.

Fatigue! They were right. It is now the new normal. Gone are the days of rakes, shovels, and hoes. Past are the enjoyments of cutting wood for the winter and sitting before a cozy fire. Vanished are the days of driving to distant destinations, as only the close and short trips are physically tolerable. Here to stay are the daily naps that enable me to do anything after the morning hours. To omit one adds more fatigue in the afternoon and a sure collapse into bed early. Now, elevators are my new friends and handrails, walls and anything else to help me remain steady are of great comfort to me. I can still think, unless tired, and type on the computer, but even my mental stamina is fatigued. My work day is now from around 8:00 a.m. till 11:00 a.m. I describe my condition to others by saying that I am a river a hundred yards wide but only half an inch deep. I do have the ability to move about but to carry anything at all is very draining. But God's grace is sufficient. There is peace in putting aside the former ways and trusting God to help you accept the new. It is not my choice or my desire, but it is where I am, and God gives me strength to live joyfully in it.

Disability is now my retirement. My heart doctor said it would be permanent due to my heart condition. But even there, God's grace shines its light. Whereas before I had no income, now I have an early retirement. I am able to give myself to the Single Mothers' Home to the extent that I can. I have freedom from the pressures of being concerned about how we will financially survive. Disability isn't enough

EARL J. SPIVEY JR.

to fully meet our needs, so I began drawing some from my retirement account and now that I have enough energy to speak, I have been given the joy of speaking a couple of times a week at a church. As a result, they provide me with enough financial help that I no longer need to withdraw funds from my retirement account. My wife and my family doctor felt it was necessary to get me handicap parking privileges. So now if I am tired, I can park close to the store or business I need to enter. I seldom use it as I want to keep my heart doing as much as it will.

Whether it is due to chemo or unrelated, I do not know. My back, which developed spinal stenosis years ago, is now much more aggravated. My muscles and joints are stiff and difficult to get moving after being in a bed or chair. Stairs are my new antagonist. But they push me to not give in and let the disability become totally disabled. It requires much more effort to move about, but there is a demonstration of grace. The strength to go beyond our natural limitations reveals an inner strength. My faith tells me that that strength is grace.

Digestion! The most visible element of chemo is the loss of hair. One of the longest lingering issues involves digestion. As the doctor explained it to me, the chemo basically kills the faster growing cells. Cancer is a fast-growing cell, and, therefore, by targeting them, you will get the cancer cells. The problem is that you also get the good fast-growing cells too. Hair is one of them but another is your digestive system. When taking chemo, your digestive system takes a major hit. That is why sores often appear in the mouth. Worse is the many other sores from your throat throughout your intestinal tract. The results are much discomfort but also nausea. So until the damage is repaired, you are battling nausea. As mentioned, the nausea is accompanied by difficulties involving the taste and salivary glands.

After chemo, some patients find their digestive system returns to normal. Others, however, only live with a new normal. Such is my case. Seldom is the nausea severe but often, I feel the return of the nagging nausea feeling that causes you to eat with great care or just avoid eating for a time. It isn't continual, just a constant return to earlier days you hoped were long gone.

I have learned to manage it without nausea pills. I will often feel the nausea creeping in and grab the candied ginger root. My wife keeps some in the pantry, and I keep some in the car. Beware, it looks a lot like candied pineapple but doesn't taste anything like it. I only made the mistake once.

I have found candied ginger to be a big help in the queasy feeling that comes from time to time. Chewing a small piece usually relieves the queasy feeling. You don't feel as comfortable eating as before but able to eat to at least help obtain nutrition. For me, it has been a continuing unwanted annoyance. Sometimes, you want to eat like a horse but have to settle for a much smaller portion. When the food settles in your stomach, you begin to sense the unsettling of your stomach. So you just stop and chew some ginger root and eat a little later when you feel your stomach will accept it.

You find that you may have to relearn what and how much to eat. Your diet is not restricted, but your tolerance has changed. You may remember the enjoyment of the foods prior to chemo, but times have changed, and no one can turn the clock back. "Give me grace, Lord," I pray. And His grace is sufficient for each day.

There are many more undesirable elements of the now daily normal life. Many experience what I am experiencing and often have more severe issues. My encouragement to you is to remember, "My grace is sufficient." Like the apostle Paul, we will not get everything we ask of God. Yet, we can be assured that God will provide all we need. If we choose to let our disabilities become disabling, then our living will be filled with hurt, anger, bitterness, and resentment. But if we choose to accept a grace only God can give us, our life will be marked by a continued forward movement and joy in that which can be experienced. We all have difficulties with which we must live. But may we all also accept a grace that will enable us to still live and not just survive or be crushed under our heavy load.

Lesson 7: Every Cross Has a Shadow

Forgive me for completing this journey with what some may consider a sad note. In all honesty, I can say that even with the shadows we will see, I really am having the greatest time of my life. My freedom from the tug of earthly things and desires has given me a much greater joy in living for a spiritual purpose. Being on disability has given me freedom to invest what I am able to do to matters unable to financially support me. My limited but better health has allowed me to do more of the significant things of life. Being free to give administration to Bethesda for Single Mothers is greatly rewarding. And my opportunity to share with others, along with God's confirmation of what I am doing, has given me a much greater enthusiasm for life. I can say this in all honesty.

So, why close with a dark note? Because the glitter and glory of being chosen as a vessel of God must be sobered with the reality that every cross has its shadows. When I think of Jesus's cross, literally and figuratively, I see much brokenness around Him. It wasn't that He wanted those around Him to suffer. It was simply a part of the cost of doing the Father's will. In less than two years after being born, Jesus's birth and recognition as Judah's promised king resulted in the death of all infant and toddler age male children in Bethlehem. When I read the story of Jesus staying in the temple, to his mother and father's nightmare, it points to a disconnecting relationship when only twelve years old. We are told in the Gospels that Jesus's mother and brothers came to take Him home, thinking he was mentally unstable. If Jesus was serious when he told a would-be follower that he literally had no place to call home, then He endured many physical hardships.

What about Mary and Joseph? The humiliation Mary endured during her pregnancy must have been crushing. Joseph came under the same humiliation when he took her as his wife. They had to make the trip to Bethlehem, start their family in a place where animals were kept, become exiles in Egypt, and finally return to those who looked condescendingly upon them. Think of the costs, struggles, and stress the couple lived under to raise our Savior. And then the ultimate pain as Mary saw Jesus beaten, mocked, and nailed to a cross. Surely, she wept in brokenness and felt all her sacrifice and love were given for nothing. Though there was great celebration at Jesus's resurrection, Mary was still to endure much heartache. What had her devotion and care for Jesus caused her with her family? While on the cross, Jesus entrusted her welfare to His disciple John. Why would not Jesus's brothers have been given that familial responsibility?

Let me walk with you through the Bible and point out some of the instruments God used and how His use of them cast shadows upon themselves and more heartbreakingly upon those around them. We can start with Abraham. To be used of God, he had to leave all of his family. He never saw any of his family again. And remember Isaac. When Abraham took him up Mount Moriah, he was tied up and lain upon an altar to be a sacrifice to prove Abraham's devotion to God. If you will survey Genesis, you will find that Abraham made at least several altars at which to worship God. Jacob, his grandson, made at least four or five. But Isaac is only credited with making one altar. It was made after God promised to bless him and place upon him the promise given to his father Abraham. God appeared to Isaac and told him not to be afraid of Him. I think that is significant. It appears to me that Isaac wanted nothing to do with an altar after he almost lost his life upon one. I wish there were more given to us about Isaac's relationship with his father. I sometimes wonder how I would respond if I witnessed my father trying to take my life in sacrifice to his God. I think the shadow of Abraham's cross fell darkly upon Isaac. How might that act of obedience have changed the relationship between Abraham and Sarah?

What about David? He was the greatest king of Judah, a mighty warrior and amazing man of organization and leadership. Yet we see that his own son sought to kill him and take over the kingdom David had built. When Absalom chased David out of Jerusalem and was finally killed, David mourned intensely at the loss of his son. It seems that David might have been a great leader, but he was a poor father. The shadow of his cross left painful family scars.

Two of Israel's greatest priests were Eli and Samuel. If you will do a little reading in 1 and 2 Samuel, you will see that they both had sad family lives. Eli's two sons were rejected by the people because they were living in open sin and were eventually killed by God's will. Samuel was brought to live with Eli when only a small boy. He followed Eli as priest over Israel. Toward the close of his life, we find that his sons abandoned Samuel's devotion to God. They were rejected as priests by God. How much of these lacking fathers is due to their devotion to being the vessel God wanted them to be? What cost of following God did these fathers pay?

Jump to the New Testament and you will find many examples of similar shadows. We know that Peter was married in a fishing business with several others and had a home by the Sea of Galilee. He later, shortly before Jesus's crucifixion, asked Jesus if giving up his family, abandoning his wife, and walking away from his business was all for naught. And then after Jesus's resurrection, we learn that Peter traveled extensively taking with him his wife but no longer with his extended family. Nothing is ever said about children and the price his devotion to Christ had upon them.

Let's consider not only the disciples. Paul's most trusted and loyal companion was Timothy. Paul met Timothy on his second missionary trip. Timothy was circumcised then left with Paul to travel much of the known world. Many hardships and heartaches were experienced. No record is ever mentioned of Timothy ever seeing his family again. The biblical records do not show Paul and his companions ever returning to Timothy's hometown.

What cost did Luke pay to go with Paul and attend to him? What struggles did early Christians endure because of their faith in Jesus Christ? Jesus made it clear when He declared that anyone who was ready to follow Him would have to put self aside, take upon himself the daily cost of dying, and follow the ways and will of Christ. Did any of His followers grasp the cost to be paid? Do you and I have any idea of how the shadow of our cross will fall upon us and those around us today?

I didn't ask for leukemia, but I did entrust myself to Christ for whatever He wished to do through me. My anticipations were for hardships and difficulties in life but not a crushing illness. As I came to believe in God's using me through leukemia, I gained a new understanding of the cost of following Christ. Let me share some of these with you and review some already shared.

The most difficult part of my journey has been the pain I continue to see in those around me. I have wept and mourned in what I see in others, especially my family, that appears to be suffering from my cross. Yet I accept that for the many preceding me and many more following me, each cross will have a shadow.

My wife has been more than faithful and caring throughout my journey. I see in her the aging that the stress and physical weight of my illness has brought upon her. Being a nurse was a huge advantage. But time after time, she was emotionally torn from her children to be by my bedside. Mile after mile, she would make the trip to the hospital over two hours away with never a complaint. She knew God would provide her with the strength and stood steady and solid time and again. After my transplant, she would often leave home before day to be at my hotel room by 7:00 a.m. to take me to the cancer center and then in the afternoon shed tears to have to leave me alone so she could return home to be with our children. Over and over, I could share the sacrifices and costs she has had to pay to go with me through this journey. And never with complaint or frustration at being my personal nurse and wife. She demonstrated a tremendous selfless love for me.

My daughter was only thirteen when I was diagnosed. She watched a strong and protecting father waste almost completely away. She had many struggles and temptations that needed the guidance and support of a loving father. Just entering high school with all its challenges, she was left to be home with family and friends most of her beginning semester. Almost every weekend was spent traveling to Charleston, sleeping in a hotel, and staying in my hospital room. Week by week, she saw my physical crumbling and felt the separation from her parents in her life. She made big steps to be independent but often in the wrong direction. She felt the guiding ropes of our time and attention slipping away. And there was also the constant questions and concerns of my not living through the experience. As I see her poor choices and grasping for another's comfort, I wonder how much comes from the shadow of my cross.

My son was a happy and active boy. He was twelve years old and full of energy. When he came each weekend, he stayed in the room with me. He, too, asked about my possible dying. He, too, witnessed the frailty of my health and uncertainty of my continued living. During the next couple of years of treatment and struggle, the active boy became a quiet and withdrawn son. He lost his athletic interest and desire to get out and attend social activities. He began to question if living had any purpose and what was the use of living if we just die and it is all taken away. It is called depression. Though improving, his introverted ways are now his sanctuary. His interest in accomplishing and achieving are absent. My wife and I pray constantly for his return to the happy and active person he was. We cry out daily for God to protect him from the dangers of depression. I often shed tears of pain as I pray for my children and see the shadow of my cross resting darkly upon them.

It would be nice to think that my medical struggles are past, but the truth is that I live under a constant dark cloud. I am presently in remission but will never be cured. The FLT3 mutation and the leukemia could be still present and just dormant reappearing at some unpredictable time sending me back into leukemia. Yes, some do live many years after their remission and transplant, but most experience short lives. I am presently in year four so I cannot celebrate being one of the 50 percent who are alive five years after treatment for at least another year. Every sore throat, every virus, and every abnormal experience leaves me with fear of leukemia's return. I have a trust in God not to deliver me from leukemia's return but for peace to walk back into death if needed. The reality is that if my leukemia returns, it will probably be for the last time. So I go wide open and as far as I can because I know this day and this week may be all I have.

As already shared, there are many limitations and weaknesses in my own shadow. The fatigue and limited ability to move about frustrates and sometimes even angers me. The continual battle with nagging medical issues is a constant burdensome weight. The trips to Charleston are now fewer and fewer, soon up to six months apart. God has given me enough strength to speak again, and I am making the most of the strength I have. I have talked about digestive issues and other related problems. There is the minor but deadening of nerves in my feet and other places that expand my limitations and inabilities. As I am typing this manuscript, I am growing frustrated by my constant mistakes on the keyboard. Time and again, I thank the Lord for the correct or return button, but never for a moment have I regretted carrying my cross. Yes, there is a shadow, but there is also joy from Christ.

Besides the physical are my mental frustrations. I often return to the days of sitting with my father. His mind was slowly fading away, and he would often reach back into his reservoir of past experiences but find them vacant. I often discover missing blocks of my memory. My wife will start talking about a past event, stop and say, "You don't remember anything about this, do you?" And she is right. I often find myself standing with people I know daily but, on this day, cannot recall their name. There is the feeling of being outside of this life. The interests other people have in daily living is of little interest to me. I feel like I am outside looking in. My changed priorities and interests are no longer in harmony with those around me. I died! I now live, but I must hurry for death will return. That is not a spiritual idea; it is my daily reality.

Perhaps one of the most painful parts of my shadow is saying good-bye to the things I have enjoyed most. For years, my closest friend and I shared a love for camping. We are old fogies and relive the colonial days when we camp. Cast iron equipment and paddling canoes were a joy we planned toward. In the coldest part of winter and hottest part of summer, we traveled down the rivers of northeastern South Carolina. Those days are gone. Too stiff to sleep on a cot, too cold-natured to bear the winter, too weak to bear the summer heat, too little stamina to paddle, and too great a risk of sickness or infection restrain me.

A few weeks ago, my camping companion came to see me. When he was leaving, I brought out all my revolutionary reenacting clothing and gear. I gave it to him to be used by any participant who didn't have clothing for the reenactments. It was painful and awkward. It was a reminder of my limitations and forever changed life.

I remember a drama I watched when a young man. The drama group was doing a play that focused on our struggles and Christ's comfort in them. One of the scenes was between an aging pastor who was being forced to resign due to his age and a noncommunicating church member in a nursing home. It was a very touching glimpse into the thinking of those unable to communicate with us. The voice speaking the thoughts of the invalid man shared an image that I especially find relevant to my life today. The subject was the aging and limitation the two older adults were experiencing. The man in his wheelchair thought in response to the pastor's heartache, "Dying is like God going through our house and turning off the lights one room after another."

Yes, I have many lights that have been turned off. I have days that the clouds of depression appear. I have many sorrows over what is no longer part of my life. But I also have peace and joy in being an instrument of the Lord. I have a freedom to use myself up in service for Christ. I have the wonder of what God has done for me and through me. I have a much greater appreciation for life's experiences and a clearer grasp of life's purpose and significance. Don't pity me or feel sorry for me. I feel that the cross I have taken and continue to carry has blessed me to do the one thing Peter did that no one else has yet to do. At Jesus's invitation, Peter climbed out of the safety of his boat and walked on water. Sure, he was carried back to the boat, but Peter is the only man in history to walk on liquified water. I feel God has given me just such a privilege. Sure, there was and will be struggles, sorrows and heartache. But there is also the amazing experience of God's closeness and greater presence because of the journey.

Thanks for taking this journey with me. May what you have read and felt along the way enrich and deepen the journey you take.

My prayer for you:

> Father, make the person reading this account more aware of your love and presence in their life. May their struggles become crosses of victory and elation as they trust in you. Grant them to experience the joy and significance you have

given me and help them see your being at work in them. Bless each reader, I ask and make your glory known to all the earth I pray. Amen.

Blessings and peace upon your journey!

Peace, comfort I give to you.

Many of you have grown disturbed of my having leukemia. Perhaps your response was like one of my dear brothers in Christ who when hearing the news cried out to God, "but God, this is one of the good guys."

As I entered the hospital on Friday (8/22) I too had many questions and much confusion as I was retested and quickly confirmed positive with leukemia. As I was taken to my room I was left to spend the night sleepless, soul-searching and eventually at peace. I turned to the Scriptures, cried out in despair and asked God for a word. It was as if I was in the Garden of Gethsemane with Christ and the Father anticipating the journey of agony. As I searched the Scriptures I was continually directed to Isaiah 53:11.

"After the suffering of his soul, he will see the light of life and be satisfied; by his knowledge my righteous servant will justify many, and he will bear their iniquities."

God reminded me of a promise I had made many years ago. A promise to be an instrument of His hand, it grew from Luke 9:23&24.

"Then he said to them all: 'If anyone would come after me, he must deny himself and take up his cross daily and follow me. For whoever wants to save his life will lose it, but whoever loses his life for me will save it.'"

Being an instrument requires that I take a cross, that I not live for me but live a life to be used up for God. God gave me the cross of parenthood, a commitment and devotion to love our two children. Irregardless of personal sacrifice or cost, but the giving of self for their good. And God reminded me of my cross to be his shepherd. The church was torn apart; great conflict damaged the body. My cross was to lay down the weapons of war, pick up the healing oil and bring back together the church family.

God gave me the cross of caregiver as He placed me beside my mother and father; to care for them in their dying years, all the while laying aside interests and self-pursuits to meet their needs.

Now a new cross. This is the cross of leukemia. It is not a curse, nor a condemnation. It is not a sign of God's forgetfulness or not being concerned. Instead it is the gift of a broken hearted Father who says to his child, "If you will carry the cross I will draw people unto me."

So I now take upon myself this cross called leukemia and neither death or life really matters. What matters is the growth of God's kingdom and the people He loves so devotedly.

As with the Apostle Paul, St. Francis of Assisi, Mother Teresa and so many others, the cross we carry is not for our own harm or good. It is instead for God's work to grow and develop. The Apostle Paul wrote in Philippians 1:12–14

"Now I want you to know, brothers, that what has happened to me has really served to advance the gospel. As a result, it has become clear throughout the whole palace guard and to everyone else that I am in chains for Christ. Because of my chains, most of the brothers in the Lord have been encouraged to speak the word of God more courageously and fearlessly."

Paul's imprisonments, beatings, sicknesses and weaknesses were all crosses God used for the Kingdom's good. So now I carry my cross and pray it is for your benefit and God's greater work in your life. I ask for prayers, not just for healing and comfort but for the outpouring of God's greater work among our human race.

Thank you for your love, your generosity, your kindness and broken compassion. I love you all as a spiritual father and friend. So be enriched by my struggles and made better because of the cross I carry.

Dictated by Earl J Spivey

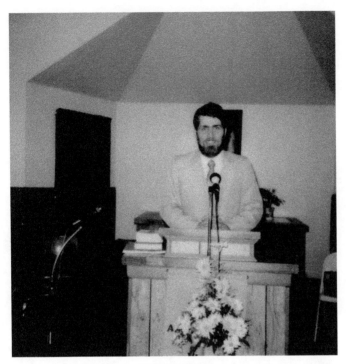

1987 Indiana

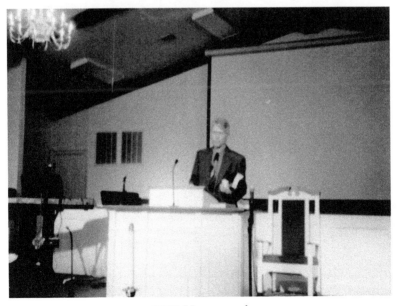

2000 Homewood

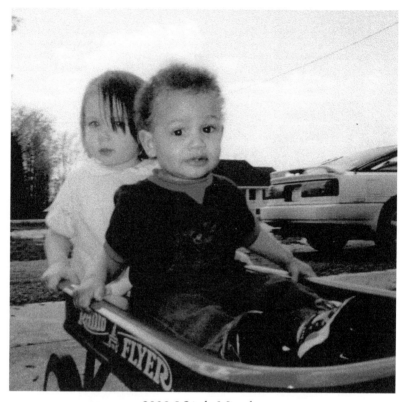

2003 2 Little Miracles

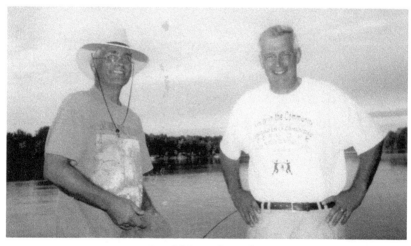

2004 Me and Denley

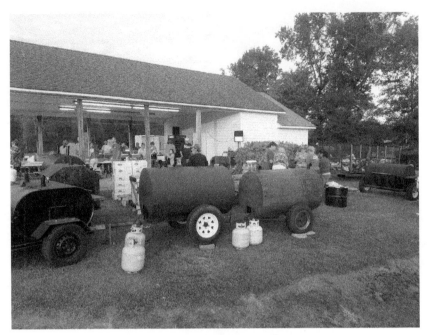

2014 Cookers at Benefit

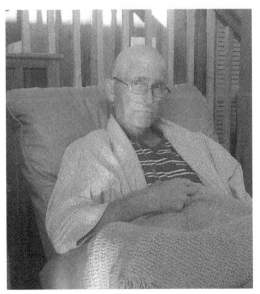

2014 Home & Barely Alive

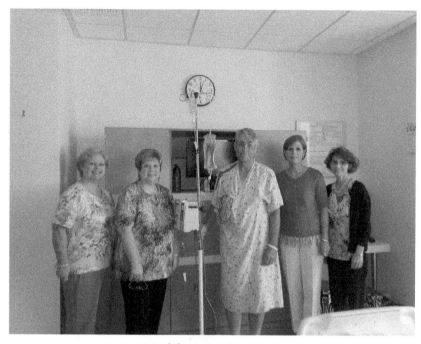

2014 Sisters at Diagnosis

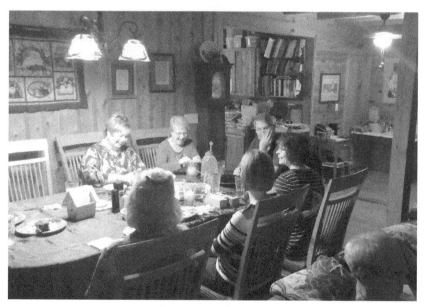

2015 Christmas Before Transplant

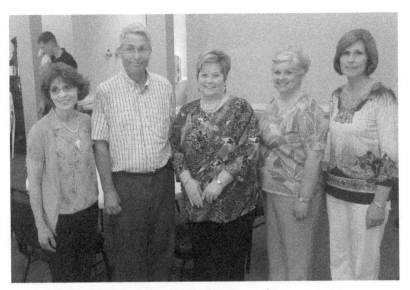

2015 Sisters before Transplant

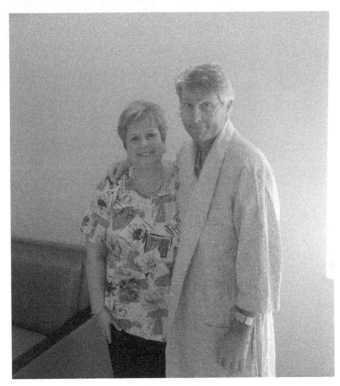

2016 Donor Sister

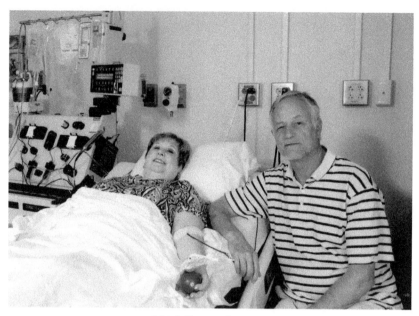

2016 Giving Support

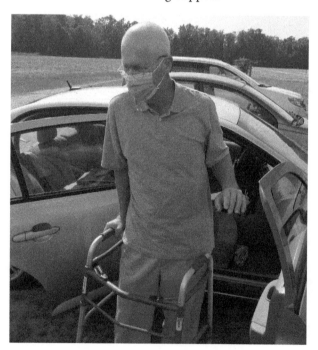

2016 Homecoming Tears

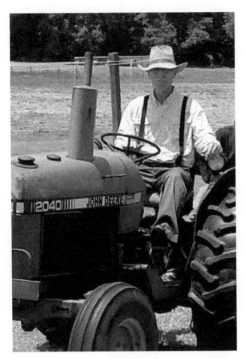

2018 A Ride of Joy

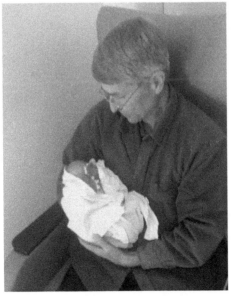

2018 Hello Grandson

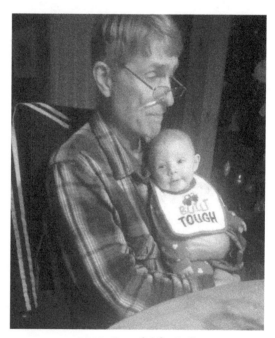

2019 Grateful for Life

About the Author

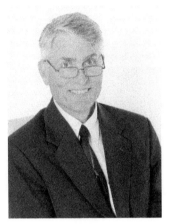

2013

Rev. Earl J. Spivey Jr. grew up on a small farm in Northeastern South Carolina. He attended Central Wesleyan College, now Southern Wesleyan University, earning a BA degree in Bible and Christian education. He attended Southeastern Baptist Theological Seminary, receiving a master's of divinity and religious education degree. Following seminary, he pastored in Indiana before returning to South Carolina. He pastored Southern Baptist Convention churches for twenty-eight years. Most were in South Carolina. He has been involved with Methodist, Presbyterian, and Episcopalian pastors and churches in ecumenical activities. He has ministered to the sick and dying, along with their families, walking with them through their disappointments and sorrows. He has a wife of thirty-eight years and two children. Being a disciple of Christ and student of the Bible has been a foundation for his life.

He is presently the executive director of Bethesda for Single Mothers. Its focus is to be a Christian community giving single mothers a place to live while completing their education and keeping their children. The goal is to enable mothers to return to society financially secure and spiritually solid. He is also completing a discipleship manual that will lead the participants to make the necessary commitments to follow and live in submission to Christ with sincerity. He is available for speaking engagements and other special events. Send your invitation and information to meadowlawnministries@gmail.com for more information.

CPSIA information can be obtained
at www.ICGtesting.com
Printed in the USA
FFHW022035101019
55476570-61278FF